THE SUICIDE PREVENTION GUIDEBOOK

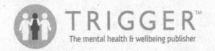

TRIGGER™
The mental health & wellbeing publisher

ABOUT THE AUTHOR

Joy Hibbins is the founder and chief executive of Suicide Crisis, a registered charity that runs suicide crisis centres. The charity's work has attracted national and international attention as a result of their zero suicide achievement. As of April 2021, they have been providing suicide crisis services for eight years, and throughout that period all clients have survived while under their care.

Their 24-hour service provides a combination of suicide crisis centres, home visits and emergency phone lines for clients under their care.

Joy set up the charity in 2012, and their first Suicide Crisis Centre opened a year later. Joy had experienced suicidal crisis herself and she felt there was a need for a different kind of crisis service. It was very important to have a highly skilled, well-trained team, but their personal qualities would be equally important: kindness and care would be at the heart of their work.

In 2016 Joy was invited to a series of meetings by the UK Government's adviser on suicide. She was asked to give a presentation about their Suicide Crisis Centre to the national advisory group on suicide prevention, which was chaired by the Government's adviser. She was subsequently invited to a meeting with the Chair of a Parliamentary Health Select Committee, where she was asked to give her opinion on the Government's new suicide prevention policy. Prior to that, she was invited to give evidence to a UK Parliamentary Select Committee, which was tasked with looking at the measures needed to prevent suicide. In the same year, the Labour Party's Shadow Minister for Mental Health visited their Suicide Crisis Centre. Joy continues to attend meetings of the UK's All Party Parliamentary Group on Suicide and Self-Harm Prevention.

In 2019 Joy was contacted by the New Zealand government, as they were drafting their new suicide prevention strategy and were wanting to learn more about the work of the charity. Further communications took place and Joy received a letter in which they commended the charity's work, described it as "inspiring" and acknowledged its contribution to "supporting other work across the world".

Joy has always felt it important that the charity remains fully independent. The charity receives no government or statutory funding. It is funded primarily by small grants and by donations from the public.

In November 2018, Joy received the Janey Antoniou award for "an outstanding contribution to addressing stigma and improving the lives of people affected by mental illness".

In January 2019, she was named in the Queen's New Year Honours List for "services to vulnerable people".

The author's royalties for this book are being donated to Suicide Crisis.

THE SUICIDE PREVENTION GUIDEBOOK

How to Support Someone Who is Having Suicidal Feelings

Joy Hibbins

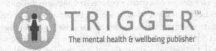

TRIGGER™
The mental health & wellbeing publisher

This edition published in 2023 by Trigger Publishing
An imprint of Shaw Callaghan Ltd

UK Office
The Stanley Building
7 Pancras Square
Kings Cross
London N1C 4AG

US Office
On Point Executive Center, Inc
3030 N Rocky Point Drive W
Suite 150
Tampa, FL 33607
www.triggerpublishing.com

A CIP catalogue record for this book is available upon request from the British Library
ISBN: 9781837963799
Ebook ISBN: 9781837963805

Typeset by Lapiz Digital Services

To my parents, with love and thanks for their constant support. And to all the clients who we have been privileged to support at our Suicide Crisis Centres – thank you for the difference you make to the world.

IF YOU ARE IN CRISIS

If you are in crisis, please call your doctor or a mental health or crisis service straight away.

If you are at immediate risk of suicide, call emergency services or go to the Emergency Department of your local hospital.

National telephone helplines

There are national suicide prevention helplines in many countries, and these provide excellent support in times of crisis.

UK and Ireland: The Samaritans on 116 123

USA: National Suicide Prevention Lifeline on 1-800-273-8255. From 2022, it will change to a three-digit number: 988.

Canada: Canada Suicide Prevention Helpline on 1-833-456-4560. There are plans to change this to a three-digit number: 988.

Australia: Lifeline on 13 11 14

New Zealand: "Need to talk?" on 1737

Your life is precious. Please seek help.

"I feel very lucky to have discovered Joy's work. I was looking for a clinical approach where people in a suicidal crisis are supported in a truly open-hearted, humane and compassionate way, as equals, which we could learn from as professionals.

Joy and the Suicide Crisis Centre have found a way to provide exactly this, and I've been seriously impressed by the service they have developed. Their methods incorporate the continuity and compassion of a good therapeutic relationship with a tenacious, proactive approach in a way that really meets people's needs in their darkest hours.

As a professional I have already learnt a lot from Joy's talks and writing, but there is a need for more. I regularly hear from carers, friends and families that they feel ill-equipped to support their loved ones in their times of need and this book will fill this important gap by offering skills and understanding that can be applied widely."

Dr Deborah Dover MBChB MRCPsych BSc (Hons)
Deputy Medical Director, Consultant Psychiatrist and Suicide Prevention Lead, Barnet, Enfield and Haringey (London) Mental Health NHS Trust

"Joy's work has become my go-to place for sound ideas, wisdom and practical guidance on suicide prevention. It comes from personal and crisis support experience, and it goes to the heart of good practice. Her work demonstrates how human connection, caring presence and building relationships of trust have to be at the centre of any response to crisis.

There is much that healthcare services need to learn about putting these principles into practice from the experience of the Suicide Crisis Centre. We know that brief interactions and "risk checklists" will not create the safety to allow expression of, and protection from, suicidal thoughts and impulses. But rarely are we shown how an alternative compassionate response can be built in practice into a crisis service. This is what Joy's work has done."

Professor David Mosse FBA FAcSS
Chair, Haringey Suicide Prevention Group
Core Member, The Alliance of Suicide Prevention Charities
Support After Suicide Partnership Leadership Team

FOREWORD

By Dr Gideon Felton MRCPsych LRCP
MD MSc BSc (Hons)

Advising psychiatrist within the charity Suicide Crisis

I became aware of the Suicide Crisis charity in 2013 during its early years and was keen to learn more about how it worked, especially in terms of how the charity had been able to listen and respond to the needs of individuals in crisis, placing them at the core of its values. This, for me, is one of the key reasons for the success of the charity.

I was honoured to be invited onto the charity's board of directors later in 2013 and my role has been that of advising psychiatrist for the past seven years.

Psychiatric services have always faced a difficult challenge when providing care for an individual who has reached such a crisis point where they believe that ending their own life seems the only option available. At the time of a crisis, it can be extremely difficult for conventional mental health services to understand the mental processes of the affected individual, with the likely result being that "safe" rather than optimal care gets provided.

Within traditional psychiatric services, I have sometimes felt there has been a disparity – that almost reached a chasm status – between the needs of patients, and the services we, as psychiatrists, have been commissioned to provide. The only way to bridge this disparity is to provide maximal opportunity for people in need (and their families) to express themselves and be heard, so that individual needs can be recognized and understood. Suicide Crisis provides this opportunity, enabling psychiatric practice to adapt and improve accordingly.

The Suicide Crisis charity has embedded lived experience knowledge and ethos into its daily work, and this means that their team members are in a strong position to understand a crisis. Gaining this understanding of someone in crisis is key to being able to provide help and support.

My own practice has improved exponentially as a result of wisdom garnered through my involvement with the charity.

This book gives many examples of the methods Suicide Crisis uses and adapts them for wider use. By sharing their ethos further, it is my hope that this could improve mental health practice internationally, as well as offering support to those in need.

PROLOGUE

By Allan Fawlk, a former client of Suicide Crisis

"You remain in my pocket for life – supporting, guiding and aiding my recovery." Allan

In 2013 a life-changing experience led to my falling into crisis and developing suicidal thoughts. I found Suicide Crisis by chance. Joy was talking about the Suicide Crisis Centre on a TV news programme. I sent a short email, and I received a reply almost immediately. That was the start of my journey with them.

By the time I visited the Centre, the team were aware of my situation and from the moment I entered, I was treated with extreme care, understanding and kindness. My counsellor had a warmth which filled the room, making it safe to talk. Professionally and with great care and empathy, she led me to voice my thoughts and feelings. Slowly, we started to walk my path together.

The Suicide Crisis Centre became my sanctuary and my safe haven. The team was determined to save my life. They were fighting with me for my survival.

My counsellor was safely in my pocket protecting me until our next contact.

They gave me the professional help and support to aid my recovery. They helped me to rebuild my self-esteem, my value and worth. They helped me re-establish my purpose.

In between the face-to-face sessions – which could take place every day if I needed them – I was encouraged to stay connected to the team via phone, email and texts.

To this day, I keep Suicide Crisis tucked safely in my pocket. Everything I learned there I carry with me.

They are an emergency service that saves lives.

Men often find it very hard to talk about their feelings, including their suicidal feelings. The staff at Suicide Crisis recognize this, and they give you time, build trust, and reassure you, allowing you to fall gently into their care.

It would be good to have such a service in every city and town, but meanwhile, this book can teach you how to help others yourself. A must-read that can save a life: a friend or relative of yours, or maybe even your own.

CONTENTS

INTRODUCTION

Your Role in Helping Someone to Survive:
What You Bring to This

Firstly, thank you so much for wanting to be there for someone who is having suicidal thoughts. Your involvement and support can make such a difference. I have written this book to provide a guide for you on that journey – to support and encourage you as well as give you important skills and knowledge.

It is very understandable if you feel apprehensive, and perhaps some self-doubt, especially if you have never supported anyone who is having suicidal thoughts before. You may feel: "Am I equipped to do this?" You have so much to offer them. The very fact that you care, you are there for them, and you want to help, can make such a difference to someone who is having suicidal thoughts.

You may already have a lot of experience of supporting someone in suicidal crisis. I have tried to include information in this book that is relevant for people who are already very knowledgeable, as well as for people who are having their first experience of supporting someone.

I run a charity that provides suicide crisis centres, where we offer predominantly face-to-face support. As I will explain later in the book, what we *see* can be just as important as

1

what we *hear*, especially when we are assessing someone's suicide risk.

We provide a combination of suicide crisis centres (which our clients can visit), home visits and emergency phone lines for clients under our care. This wraps a safety net around them, giving them more ways to access our care and stay connected with us, and giving us more ways to reach and protect them.

As of April 2021, there has never been a suicide of a client under our care, whether they have been under our care for a period of days, weeks or months. But when I set up this charity in 2012, I didn't have a "zero suicide ambition". My approach was simply that "we will do everything we can for each person, to help them to survive". That is still the approach that we take every day.

If you have never supported anyone who has had suicidal thoughts before, it may help to remember that all of us started as beginners at one time. Although I have now spent many years supporting people in suicidal crisis, I can still remember what it was like, before I had any training at all.

I remember my very first training course in suicide prevention. We were asked to take part in a powerful role play exercise. It helped me to understand something very important – that we are all far more equipped to help someone in crisis than we realize, even before any kind of training. Although the situation involved helping a stranger, the things I learned are equally important when supporting a friend or family member.

We had to enact a situation where we were out on a walk. Suddenly, we came across a person who was standing in a location of imminent risk, where they could end their life in seconds.

We were asked how we might respond in that situation, even before we had started the professional training. I remember feeling daunted and ill-equipped to help. It was such a high-risk situation. We all fell silent. It was at that point that the trainer started to play the role of the person who was at imminent risk. Suddenly it started to feel very real, and we found ourselves responding to the situation that was unfolding. I instinctively started to try to help – because I cared and was concerned. I didn't want any harm to come to this vulnerable stranger who was suffering and in emotional pain. My instinctive reaction was to use a gentle approach – approaching very gradually with a soft voice, so as not to alarm the person. Somehow I found the words to use while we waited for the emergency services to arrive, which are of course trained to work in these situations.

What I was able to convey to the stranger was that I cared, and that I was concerned for them. Their life mattered to me. I did that by the very fact that I approached them and was trying to help. My actions *showed* them that, as much as my words did. And I wanted to get help for them. For most of us, this will be our instinctive reaction when faced with someone who is at risk of ending their life.

Your care and kindness can have such a powerful effect when someone is having thoughts of suicide or is at imminent risk of ending their life.

This role play exercise was so helpful in showing us that we already had some of the qualities we needed to help someone at the point of suicide.

As well as providing you with practical skills to help you support someone who is having suicidal thoughts, this book provides you with information to help you understand more about suicidal feelings and their complexity. By having a deeper of knowledge of why someone might be experiencing suicidal thoughts, you'll be even more equipped to help them. The book also dispels some of the myths about suicide, because these myths and misconceptions can create barriers to helping someone.

If you have lived experience of suicidal crisis yourself, this will be so valuable and will equip you so well to support someone else. I know that my own lived experience of having been in suicidal crisis has made such a powerful difference. It brings an additional dimension to my work – a deeper level of understanding, knowledge and empathy – alongside my professional training. Lived experience has a profound influence on our services and the way that we work. It is at the heart of what we do, and permeates all aspects of our services.

Each year, we hear deeply concerning statistics about the number of deaths by suicide. The World Health Organization estimates that around 800,000 people die by suicide every year.[1]

The American Foundation for Suicide Prevention confirmed that, on average, 132 Americans died by suicide each day in 2020.[2]

In 2019, the UK's Office for National Statistics' (ONS) annual release showed that 5,691 deaths by suicide were registered in England and Wales in that year.[3] They were: 5,691 parents, siblings, sons or daughters, partners, cousins, friends, work colleagues or neighbours to many thousands more grieving individuals. Around three quarters of the registered deaths by suicide were men. 4,303 men died by suicide in that year, and 1,388 women.

When you read these statistics, it's important to remember that your female family member, friend or work colleague may be just as much at risk of suicide, though. It's about the person you have in front of you and their individual level of risk. The ONS statistics for 2019 showed an increase in the number of deaths by suicide of women, particularly young women aged 16 to 25.

The information in this book is designed to help you to support someone you know. You may be reading it to help someone who you think (or know) is in crisis. Or perhaps you want to be prepared, so that you can support someone who may need you in the future – whether that is a family member, friend, work colleague, neighbour or someone you know from a sports club or through your social connections.

In sharing techniques in this book to help you support someone in crisis, I would never want you to feel that you carry the responsibility for their survival. It is important to involve professionals, who can intervene and provide a different kind of help. I would not want you to feel alone on this journey. There are doctors, nurses, suicide crisis workers, psychiatric clinicians and other professionals who are trained to help and support people during a period of crisis. I will refer to them again later in the book, and I'll explain which professionals and services to involve at different stages.

It can help to think of yourself as being part of the person's support network – an important part. Your involvement can make a significant difference. Remember that you are already bringing something very powerful, even before you start reading this book to learn more about how to help someone in crisis. You bring love and care, and you genuinely want to help.

PART 1

UNDERSTANDING
A SUICIDAL CRISIS

1

YOUR FEELINGS ABOUT SUICIDE AND FIRST REACTIONS

The feelings we hold about suicide can be very complex. Our previous life experiences can influence what we think about it, and how we react when we know or suspect that someone is having suicidal thoughts.

We may react in a range of different ways at this point, in terms of our thoughts or behaviour. All of these different responses are very understandable. They originate from caring deeply about the person who is struggling with suicidal thoughts.

The aim of this chapter is to help you understand why you may be having these feelings and reactions. Some of these different feelings and reactions can create a barrier to helping your friend or loved one, and so I will show you some of the ways you can be supported through them, or helped to move beyond them.

FEAR OF LOSING THEM

This can be so painfully acute – the fear that the person will take their own life. For some of us, it is a constant underlying fear throughout the period in which we are supporting them. It is so important that someone is there for *you* at this time, so that you are able to share your fear and feelings. That "someone" may be a friend or indeed, a professional.

We provide suicide crisis centres for people at risk of suicide, but we often receive calls or visits from family members or friends of a person who is at risk. They will call to share vital information about their loved one, but as they continue to talk, we can hear the pain in their voices. We spend time talking to them about their feelings, because it matters that they can release and express such painful emotions. There are times when I have simply held them in my arms. It is important that they do not feel alone in this situation.

Sometimes carers call us for advice about a particular crisis situation and that is so important, too – knowing they can call someone for guidance. I would urge anyone caring for someone in this situation to always remember that you can call a crisis service to ask for advice. If you don't have a suicide crisis centre in your area, then you can call your local community psychiatric crisis team, or your national suicide prevention helpline to ask for advice. The numbers of some national helplines are at the beginning and end of this book.

FEAR OF "SAYING THE WRONG THING"

Understandably, when supporting someone who is having thoughts of ending their life, you may be afraid that you will say something that "makes things worse".

However, if the person you are supporting knows that you care for them and are doing everything you can to help them, it is *very* unlikely that you will accidentally say something that will be destabilizing.

If you do accidentally say something you think may be unhelpful, they are hearing it in the wider context of a person who would do anything to help protect their life at that point.

The care and support that you are providing is helping the person immeasurably, and it far outweighs any unfortunate comments you may inadvertently make.

> By caring and being there for that person, you are providing one of the most important protective factors against suicide.

And if you are so worried about "saying the wrong thing" that you find yourself saying very little, then please know that your silent presence speaks volumes. Just being there with them sends the powerful message: *"I am here for you."*

You can of course share your fear with the person you are supporting. For example: "I will do whatever I can to help. And if I get it wrong, or say the wrong thing, please tell me – because I would never want to do anything to upset you in any way."

WITHDRAWING FROM THE PERSON WHO IS AT RISK

It may be too painful to contemplate that a friend or a loved one is in crisis, or that we may lose them to suicide. As a result, you may become more distant, because it is all too painful. It feels unbearable to see them suffering, so you withdraw. You may avoid them.

It is because you care so much, and it is so hard to see them in pain. All of this is understandable. Give yourself time and space to start to come to terms with what is happening to your loved one. Talk to people – family, friends and professionals – about how painful this is, and how hard it is for you. This will help you feel more able to reconnect with your friend or loved one.

DENIAL

"This cannot be happening." Again, your mind is struggling to come to terms with the reality of the situation. You cannot bear to think that you might lose them, and so a part of your mind is unable to accept that they are in suicidal crisis. This can happen, particularly in the early stages. This early phase of denial often passes of its own accord but if not, talking to professionals can help enormously. There is more information about accessing help from professionals in Chapter 17.

MINIMIZING THE SITUATION

"It can't be that bad." "He/she will be okay." Our mind naturally reverts to the "least worst-case scenario".

It is natural to try to play down what is happening rather than seeing the reality. However, it is important for your friend or loved one that you recognize and acknowledge the extent of their emotional pain and suffering, and their risk.

Later in the book, I'll help you focus on the words they are actually saying – the reality of their situation. I'll also show you how you can "reflect back" what they are saying, to show them that you understand the depth of their pain, and their risk.

ANGER

We may feel anger because they are thinking of leaving their loved ones. "How could they think of leaving us/their family in this way?" We may find it particularly hard to understand this if we haven't felt suicidal ourselves. I'll explain in Chapter 3 that the person in suicidal crisis is not thinking as they usually would. It can help to realize that they are not themselves at the present time. Their thinking is usually being influenced either by high levels of distress and emotional pain, or by a mental health condition such as depression, or post-traumatic symptoms.

COMPARISON

We may feel anger for a different reason – because we have been through something similar, and we got through it. Thoughts might include: "I have been through similar things and I have never felt suicidal." "I have been through worse than that and I have never once felt like ending my life." I'll explain in the next few chapters that a suicidal crisis is complex. It is rarely just one thing that leads a person to want to end their life. It is usually a combination of many different factors that leads someone to be particularly vulnerable at this time.

GUILT

"Is it my fault that they are in suicidal crisis? Was it something I did or didn't do?" It can be heartbreaking to hear a parent of a grown-up child say this. I have heard parents of some of our clients say it, when they call us to ask for advice. They wonder if it was something they should have done differently when raising them. Did they do something that made their loved one more vulnerable to a suicidal crisis?

Every time a parent has said this, it has been so clear to me that they have been a deeply loving and caring parent. I have explained this to them: "By loving and caring for them in the way that you did, you gave them the best possible start – and the best protection against suicide. Love and care are profoundly protective against suicide."

If you are struggling with feelings of guilt, I would urge you to read Chapter 3. I hope it will help you to understand more about the reasons why someone may experience suicidal crisis – and how very complex it is.

IN SUMMARY

If you do recognize that you are experiencing some of the feelings and reactions touched upon in this chapter, please be reassured that they are all natural human responses to a situation that profoundly challenges us as individuals – the knowledge or belief that someone we know and care about may want to take their own life.

2

WHAT WE MEAN BY "FEELING SUICIDAL": THE COMPLEXITY OF SUICIDAL FEELINGS

The phrase "feeling suicidal" is widely understood to mean that someone is having thoughts that they want to end their life. But "feeling suicidal" is complex and it includes a range of different feelings, and there are different levels of risk within it.

Even though the feelings are complex, this doesn't mean that only professionals can help someone. You can help in so many ways. The purpose of this chapter is to increase your knowledge and understanding of suicidal feelings. *By understanding more, you will be even more equipped to be able to help.*

WHAT "FEELING SUICIDAL" CAN ACTUALLY MEAN

"Feeling suicidal" does not always mean that someone wants to die. For many people, when they talk about wanting to end their life, they want *the deep emotional pain they are experiencing to end.* A combination of events and circumstances in their life have led them to feel a level of emotional pain and suffering that feels unbearable at this point. They desperately want it to stop.

It's so important that we do our best to help them to see there are other ways to help alleviate this intense pain. Being cared for and supported by empathic individuals – including professionals – is such a vital part of this, until an individual reaches a place where they are able to contemplate living again. We have supported so many hundreds of clients at our Suicide Crisis Centres who have experienced the most intense emotional pain, who have lived through harrowing and heartbreaking circumstances, and who are now living highly meaningful lives. Now, they want to live, and are glad they have survived, even though they could never have imagined feeling this way while in the depths of their suicidal crisis.

Some people feel trapped in a situation or by circumstances, and they are struggling to see that there are other ways to escape their situation, apart from suicide. So in this case, their thoughts of suicide can be about desperately wanting to *escape* something, rather than about wanting to die. Emotional distress or high levels of psychological stress can make it hard to think clearly and to see other ways forward out of a situation. Talking to friends, family and especially professionals can help enormously, because they can look at a situation more objectively and help them to see that there are other routes forward.

For many people, their thoughts of suicide are about not feeling able to live the life they have currently, rather than actually wanting to die.

It is usually a smaller number of people who actually want to die – in the sense of wanting not to exist, rather than wanting to escape profound emotional pain or circumstances. But it can sometimes be hard for the person to make this distinction.

The reasons why someone feels suicidal are so individual, and I will explain more about this in the next chapter.

Here, I'm going to explain a little more about how the phrase "feeling suicidal" can include different levels of intensity and risk.

Some people experience a progression from passive thoughts at first, to more active thoughts, and for some people, this progresses further from "thoughts" to "wanting to act on those thoughts", and then to "intending to act on those thoughts", and planning to end their life. Not everyone goes through these different stages. And you can help at every stage, including when someone is planning to end their life.

PASSIVE THOUGHTS OF WANTING TO DIE

This means that someone wishes they were dead, but they are not having thoughts of actually ending their own life. For example, they talk about wishing that they could "go to sleep and not wake up". They wish something would happen that causes them to die prematurely. But this would not be by their own hand.

It's important that they get help and support to alleviate their emotional pain, and to prevent them from deteriorating further and developing more active thoughts. As well as providing your support, you can encourage them to talk to their doctor or another professional.

ACTIVE THOUGHTS ABOUT SUICIDE

When we talk about "active thoughts", it means that someone wants to end their own life.

The suicidal thoughts may be fleeting at first. Perhaps they only have the thoughts from time to time. But these can become much more frequent and persistent.

There are many things that can prevent them from going any further than having thoughts about suicide. There are lots of things that can prevent their suicidal thoughts from escalating to the point where they have an intention to end their life. They may still be able to think of many reasons for staying alive, at this stage. Some people will actually say: "I would never take my own life, though", and then they explain why not – listing their reasons for continuing to live.

Professionals call these "protective factors" – the things in someone's life that are protecting them against suicide. These are specific to the individual person. It's still important to get professional help at this stage from suicide crisis services, doctors or mental health services, though – because this can change. It is possible that they can deteriorate as the days or weeks go by. For example, if they are depressed, they can descend deeper into depression and lose sight of their reasons for living. Depression can change a person's thinking, as I will explain in the next chapter. Or events can happen in their life that make them feel more overwhelmed, or which cause them to deteriorate further.

If they are struggling to see reasons for living, they can be helped to find them. There are ways you can help them to reconnect with things that are meaningful for them, or help them to find meaning in their life; I will explain how to do this in this book.

Your care and support, and professional help, can also become additional protective factors. The support of friends, family, community and professionals is known to help protect against suicide.

SUICIDAL INTENT

For some people, their suicidal thoughts escalate and they start to think about *how* they would end their life. Some people deteriorate further still, and start to have *suicidal intent* (intending to end their life). They may then start to plan to end their own life. But they can absolutely be helped, and it is important that they get professional help immediately, as I will explain in Chapters 6 and 7. It is possible to intervene, help and protect their life at each stage – even if they are at the point of suicide.

EXPLAINING THE TERM "SUICIDAL CRISIS"

In this book, I sometimes use the phrase "suicidal crisis". The phrase can be used to describe someone who is contemplating suicide; it includes someone who is having suicidal thoughts or someone who has suicidal intent. So the phrase describes quite a wide spectrum of intensity and risk. When someone is starting to deteriorate and their thoughts of suicide become stronger, they are descending deeper into crisis. If they continue to deteriorate to the point where they have an intention to end their life, their crisis has escalated further. We provide suicide crisis centres and they are open to anyone, whether they are having thoughts of ending their life, or have a strong intention to end their life. "Suicide crisis" has to be a broad, inclusive term.

It's important to emphasize that everyone is an individual and their experience of suicidal feelings will be different. Their paths into and through suicidal crisis will be unique to them, too.

If someone wants to end their life, in my opinion it is a crisis, whether they are having suicidal thoughts or a strong intention to end their life.

IN SUMMARY

As I have emphasized throughout this chapter, it's possible to intervene and help, even when someone is at the point of suicide. In Chapter 7, I will show you the right questions to ask to establish an individual's risk of suicide, and how immediate the risk is. And throughout Part 2, How to Help, I will show you how you can help support them through their crisis.

IN SUMMARY

3

UNDERSTANDING WHAT MAY LEAD TO A SUICIDAL CRISIS

The reasons why someone experiences a suicidal crisis are complex. It is rarely caused by a single event. It is usually a combination of many different factors. However, a single event may be a final trigger for a suicidal crisis, at a time when someone is already vulnerable.

The more you understand about what has led your friend or family member to develop suicidal thoughts, the more you can support and help them.

I'm going to explain briefly the experience of one of our clients, so that you can see some of the different factors involved in the lead-up to his suicidal crisis.

A COMBINATION OF MANY DIFFERENT FACTORS: LIFE EVENTS

John explained to us that his wife had left him suddenly and unexpectedly. It was a massive shock to him: "She told me she was leaving me and walked out that same day. I didn't see any signs that it was going to happen. She said she had met someone else."

If you had met John at that time, you might have assumed that he developed suicidal thoughts because his wife had left him. But it was much more complex than that.

It became clear that John had experienced two traumatic deaths in his family several years before. These were sudden and unexpected deaths. He suppressed his own emotions and his own pain at the time of both deaths. He took care of everyone else in the family instead. He focused on them. He supported them and comforted them. He did not talk about his own feelings of loss. The pain of both deaths remained locked inside him. He did not have the chance to grieve for either of his relatives.

All these experiences – the recent loss of his wife, and the previous loss of family members through death – had something in common. They all involved the deeply painful loss of a loved one, which happened suddenly and unexpectedly. *As a result, his wife's sudden departure triggered powerful memories and feelings about these two previous sudden, painful losses.* He said that he felt he was now experiencing the pain of all these losses at once – his wife leaving him, and the earlier deaths of family members. He was also now feeling all the complex emotions that had been buried – including intense guilt, which is so often a part of traumatic grief. His suffering was immense at this time.

Suicidal feelings arise most often from emotional pain and suffering which becomes unbearable.

Events from the past – even many years in the past – can be a factor in someone's suicidal crisis. It is often about more than recent events.

John was also vulnerable in other ways at the time of his wife leaving him. He had been seriously ill for many months, and he was physically and psychologically affected by that. His inner reserves had been depleted and so it was much harder to cope with a sudden distressing event. He was more fragile because of his very recent illness. He had become unable to work because of his illness, and his illness had affected him physically in many ways.

It is likely, from what he told us, that he was already depressed at the time his wife left him. Depression was another factor that left him much more vulnerable to a suicidal crisis.

As you can see, John was being affected by many different experiences including the ending of his marriage, his feeling that he had lost his place/role in the family, the deaths of family members from years ago, trauma and suppressed grief, being isolated and feeling alone, the impact of physical illness, the loss of his job, and a decline in his mental health.

For some people, the factors contributing to suicidal crisis don't just include past or current events. They can also include the anticipation of future events.

The future event might be something frightening or distressing such as a court case, or it might be a major life change such as starting university. I'll explain more about this in Chapter 5.

OUR INDIVIDUAL COPING STYLES

There were a number of factors that led to John's suicidal crisis, but his *individual coping style* also had an impact. He didn't talk to family or friends, and this left him isolated and alone in his suffering.

We all learn to cope differently with major life events and adverse experiences. We sometimes learn a particular way of coping at a very young age. This may be because of cultural expectations, or the way we are brought up, or because we experience difficult life events in childhood.

Some of us have learned to "suppress and carry on". This means that we suppress our own pain and emotions during major life events, and continue as usual. We don't talk about our feelings. We bury them inside ourselves, just as John did.

Sometimes we develop this approach because we instinctively think of other people first. *We focus on their needs, not our own.* We are the person who helps and supports everyone else during a family crisis.

Another reason for "suppressing" is because of cultural or gender expectations, particularly some traditional expectations about how men should react to adverse events. Some men were brought up not to show emotion, and not to appear vulnerable.

This often means that *we have never learned to ask for help*. When we start to struggle, we just keep going. If we could reach out and talk, and ask for help at this early stage, it could prevent a further deterioration. This coping style can make us more vulnerable in the longer term. Learning to share our emotions and talk about emotional pain is an important part of our mental wellbeing.

Another of our clients, Gemma, had also learned to "suppress and carry on". In her early childhood, there were a number of deaths in her wider family. This led her to become very self-reliant at a young age. She felt that she could not rely on other people too much because they might die, too. Her self-reliant coping style led her to become very independent, but it also meant that she did not learn to ask for help during difficult times. In the longer-term, this made her more vulnerable, just like John.

HOW WE THINK DIFFERENTLY DURING A SUICIDAL CRISIS: DEPRESSION

Many people who experience suicidal crisis are depressed or are being impacted by some other mental health condition. Sometimes it is obvious that someone is depressed – you can see lots of signs that they are feeling very low in mood. But it is not always so obvious. They may be trying very hard to mask it. Many people who are depressed work very hard to present to the world as if they are okay.

Depression can temporarily change the way that someone thinks about life. It can make them think that there is no hope.

It is as if it throws a dark veil over everything. *It can also change the way someone thinks about themselves.* They stop seeing themselves as they really are. They may start to believe that they have no worth. Over time, they may start to feel that it would be better if they did not exist at all. Of course, none of this is true – it is how depression temporarily distorts and changes someone's thinking. They may start to see themselves as a negative presence in the world, or a burden to others: they struggle to believe that they have any good qualities at all. I'll explain later in the book how you can help and support someone who is thinking in this way.

Many people who are depressed say it feels like being in a "dark tunnel". It can be so hard for them to see an end to it. All they can see is darkness stretching ahead of them. For someone who is depressed, that may be exactly how they see the future – simply more darkness ahead. We can see that things will change for them – that it will not always be as it is now. But it can be so hard for them to believe it.

It is important that we emphasize that it does have an end, and that we keep reinforcing this. I remember Mark, one of our clients, used to ask me regularly: "There is light at the end, isn't there? I can't see it anymore." It was important to him to regularly have this reassurance that his depressive episode would end. Now, several months later, he is feeling so much better and is planning for his future.

Depression is an illness and it's important to emphasize this. It is a treatable illness. Their doctor can refer them for treatment and help, including talking therapy, which the UK's National Institute for Health and Care Excellence (NICE) recommends for depression.[4]

The tunnel metaphor also helps to explain the kind of restricted vision and restricted world someone might have when they are depressed. Everything and everyone they care about is outside the tunnel, so they can no longer see them. It can mean that they become disconnected from the people they care about. They can start to feel more and more detached from other people, as they go deeper into the tunnel. The later chapters will explain how you can keep connected with them, and will suggest ways that you can break through the barriers depression has created around them.

THE IMPACT OF TRAUMATIC EVENTS

Traumatic events can be extremely destabilizing. They can affect us for many months, and sometimes for years. It is very important to receive the right help and support afterwards – including the right professional help. Childhood trauma can continue to affect us as adults. Trauma in adulthood can be devastating, too.

The symptoms of post-traumatic stress can lead us to keep "re-living" an event through flashbacks – images of the traumatic event keep coming into our mind. We may re-live the event in traumatic nightmares, too. These post-traumatic symptoms can feel overwhelming to some people. It can feel as though they cannot escape the original trauma.

We may feel a complex range of emotions after a traumatic event, including guilt.

Trauma often causes us to detach from other people. It can shatter our trust in people – and our trust in the world as a safe place.

Being supported is one of the most important and helpful things for an individual after traumatic events. It often takes time before the person is ready for psychological therapy or trauma-focused therapy from professionals, to help them process the events. The support they receive from friends or loved ones in the meantime can be an important part of their eventual recovery.

It's important not to try to draw detailed information out of the person about their trauma. Clinicians recommend that you do not ask questions or encourage them to talk in detail about deeply traumatic events. It could be destabilizing or re-traumatizing for them. It is psychologists or other professionals who can safely work with someone after trauma.

You can still have a vital role, though. Being there, caring, supporting – it can all be part of helping someone to rebuild trust in other people.

THE IMPACT OF HIGH LEVELS OF DISTRESS

It is not just mental illness that can temporarily change the way that we think. *High levels of distress can also affect our ability to think clearly and rationally.* It can mean that someone is not thinking as they usually would. It can also make them more impulsive. If they are highly distressed, they are *less in control of their emotions* than usual. If they are less able to control their emotions, then they *may be less able to control their actions*.

So if you are struggling to understand why someone you know is in suicidal crisis, it may help to think of it in this way:

they are not themselves at the moment. They are not acting in a way that they usually would. They are nearly always being influenced by high levels of emotional pain and distress, or mental illness (such as depression). *Sometimes these factors are not obvious – it is possible to mask depression and even severe distress.*

Someone who has recently been in suicidal crisis may express guilt about things they have done during that period of crisis. They sometimes tell me that they feel remorse for things they have said – especially things they have said to the people they love. I usually explain to them that they were in crisis at the time. When you are in crisis, it is often a time of internal chaos. Your thinking may be chaotic at the time. And this means you may act very differently from usual. Clients will often say to me, "That is not who I am – that is not me. I am not someone who shouts or says things like that to the people I love." It is very often the case that a suicidal crisis makes a person act in a way that they never usually would.

Severe distress is just as likely to be expressed in anger as in tearful sorrow. Anger can be a particular risk factor. It can increase a person's risk of suicide, because of the loss of control they may experience. In Chapter 14, I will explain more about supporting someone who is angry and in crisis.

MENTAL ILLNESS

I've already explained how depression can affect the way someone thinks. But there are other forms of mental illness that can influence how someone thinks, for example, a psychotic episode.

PSYCHOTIC EPISODES

A psychotic episode can happen in the context of a previously diagnosed mental health condition like schizophrenia or bipolar disorder. But the Royal College of Psychiatrists in the UK explains that it can also happen to someone after a deeply distressing major life event such as the death of a close relative.[5] We know that it can also occur after a deeply traumatic experience.

People can have very different thoughts and experiences during a psychotic episode, and not everyone will have thoughts of ending their life. The Royal College of Psychiatrists describes psychosis as "losing touch with reality".[5] Some people prefer to talk about an "altered reality". They may have unusual thoughts or experiences. They may have delusional thoughts – beliefs that are not true.

Some people who have a psychotic episode believe that they are receiving messages telling them to end their life. Or they hear voices that are telling them to end their life. It is very important that they can access psychiatric help at this point. You can help them access this via the Emergency Department of a general hospital or by calling your local crisis resolution team within psychiatric services. And while you are doing that, your caring support and your reassurance (that they will get help) will also help enormously.

The Royal College of Psychiatrists has a leaflet, Psychosis Information for Parents and Carers, which explains more about causes, symptoms and treatment.

IMPACT OF ALCOHOL OR DRUGS

Sometimes people start using alcohol or drugs to block out emotional pain – to try to blunt the painful emotions. They may also use them to try to cope with the symptoms of mental illness or trauma.

A high percentage of our clients who use alcohol or drugs started to use them to block out their post-traumatic symptoms. This includes flashbacks and "night terrors". One of our clients used to drink large quantities of alcohol every evening to try to avoid the terrifying dreams, which seemed entirely real to her, where she would re-live the traumatic events of her past. Her plan was always to drink so much that she would go into a deep sleep where she would not be awakened by her terrifying dreams. But the high levels of alcohol had a very detrimental long-term impact on her, both mentally and physically.

Using alcohol or drugs can significantly increase the risk of suicide. It affects our ability to think clearly and make the kind of decisions that we usually would. It means that *we have less control over what we do*. It can lower our inhibitions and make us more reckless, too. And it is a depressant, so it can lower our mood even more. It can make us feel more depressed.

Alcohol or drug use can contribute to suicide risk in less direct ways, too. Severe addiction can eventually lead to someone losing many of the things that are most important to their mental health and wellbeing: their relationships and social connections, their employment, and sometimes their home.

And, as I explained earlier, the addiction is usually masking a much deeper pain such as trauma. Over time, the addiction can also affect how someone feels about themselves and about life in general. I remember the words of one of our clients, in particular. He is an extremely caring and much-loved grandfather who has recently struggled with alcohol addiction. He told me: "I am no good now – no use to anyone", and "I used to be there for my grandchildren. I tried to be a role model for them. Now look at me. I am no use to anyone." *He was still the same loving, supportive, caring and protective grandfather, though.* We still saw all of those qualities in him, and we reminded him frequently of what we saw in him.

When you first start to support someone who is in crisis, you may not be aware that they are using quite large amounts of alcohol. They may have built up a tolerance to some of its effects, so they may not immediately show obvious signs of being intoxicated. However, the excess alcohol is still having a damaging effect.

You can help your friend or loved one by gently encouraging them to access local drug and alcohol recovery services. In the UK we can usually access free services, which support people in the community. Their doctor can make the referral. It's also usually possible to self-refer. You can phone the service on behalf of your friend or a loved one to find out what they offer, especially if they feel anxious about making contact. You can find out for them what it would involve. Taking the first step toward help can feel hard. But the professionals will simply want to help. They will want to find what will work best for your friend or loved one individually. Many people who work in the services have had previous experience of using alcohol or drugs themselves, and have a deep understanding of the issues.

It is often so important that mental health services are involved as well, especially when someone is using drugs or alcohol to try to alleviate symptoms of mental illness or the effects of trauma. Mental health services can provide support until they are ready to start psychological therapy or trauma-focused therapy. I know that there can sometimes be difficulties in accessing the ongoing help from psychiatric services that your friend or family member needs, and I will explore that in Chapter 15, which is about supporting people through more than one crisis.

IN SUMMARY

As this chapter has shown, it is usually a combination of life events along with many other factors which makes someone more vulnerable to a suicidal crisis. In the next chapter, I'll help you to understand even more about suicide, by dispelling some of the myths and misunderstandings that can create barriers to helping someone.

4

MYTHS AND MISUNDERSTANDINGS ABOUT SUICIDE

There is a lot of misinformation about suicide and this can influence your thinking and make it harder for you to give someone the most effective help. In this chapter, I'm going to address and dispel the myths, to help increase your understanding of suicide and create the foundations for you to provide the best possible help you can.

Myths can stop people from asking for help, because they feel they won't be taken seriously, or that they will be judged, misunderstood or treated in a negative way if they tell someone that they are having suicidal thoughts. The myths help perpetuate stigma and silence.

MYTH 1

"A genuinely suicidal person won't ask for help. They will just go off quietly and end their life."

This myth feeds into the idea that if someone has genuine strong suicidal intent, they will go and take their own life without telling anyone, so that there is no opportunity for anyone to help. It gives the impression that there isn't much (or anything) that you can do to help someone who is "genuinely suicidal".

In reality, many people who go on to end their lives ask for help for their suicidal thoughts at some point, or they tell someone or give other indications that they are at risk of suicide.

When someone asks for help, you may only have a short window of opportunity in which to do so. Their willingness to seek help may fluctuate. If they are depressed, their depression may deepen as the days pass – and their suicide risk may increase, too. As they become more depressed, they may withdraw from the world and stop seeking help. So it is vital that we try to help them while we can, because they might withdraw and stop asking in a few days' or a few weeks' time.

Sometimes, there is only a very small part of them that is trying to survive. You sometimes hear counsellors explaining to their client that they are trying to "work with that small part of them which is trying to stay alive".

In 2017-18, Suicide Crisis undertook research into deaths by suicide in Gloucestershire, UK.[6] This research found that most people who took their own life revealed their suicidal thoughts to someone in the weeks before their death, whether it was their doctor, a psychiatric professional, a friend or a family member.

The fact that someone tells you they are feeling suicidal does not mean that they are less at risk of taking their own life, as I explain below. It is so important to recognize their risk and respond.

MYTH 2

"People who talk about suicide don't do it."

This is similar to the previous myth. In fact, someone who is at risk of suicide may well "talk about it", and draw your attention to their risk. Within days, their willingness to talk and reach out for help may have evaporated, and they may end their life. That is why it is so important to hear them and recognize their risk of suicide, so that you can make sure that they get help and support. Chapter 7 will guide you through direct questions to ask about suicide.

MYTH 3

"People who make casual remarks about feeling suicidal are not genuine."

Sometimes a person may make quite casual remarks about wanting to die. It would be easy to miss the significance of these, because of the way in which they are expressed.

As part of our research into deaths by suicide in 2017-18, we attended inquests over a six-month period. Two of the individuals who died had made casual remarks about suicide in the days before they died. One of them said: "I don't know why I don't just kill myself." The other said: "I might as well kill myself." Both of them referred to a particular method of suicide.

Understandably, friends and family members might not immediately recognize these remarks as a sign of increased risk. The casual nature of the remarks can give a false sense of security. Our research shows how important it is to take notice of every expression of suicidal intent, however it is expressed.

> It can be very difficult to tell friends or family members that you are having suicidal thoughts. This is why some people may say it in a casual way.

MYTH 4

"Asking about suicide may give someone the idea to do it."

Research shows that asking direct questions about suicide helps to protect someone's life, and that it does *not* put the idea into their head.

In a research study carried out in London among 443 adults in a primary care clinical setting, the findings showed no evidence that asking about suicidal thoughts increased hopelessness or made the participants think that life was not worth living.[7]

In other research in the USA, it was found that asking young people about suicidal thoughts did not increase distress or suicidality afterwards, and that there were beneficial effects for people who were showing signs of depression or had previously attempted suicide.[8]

Asking questions about suicidal thoughts gives someone the opportunity to disclose their risk. It can be very difficult for them to tell someone that they are feeling suicidal. They may want to, but they may not know how.

> Most people feel a profound sense of relief when they disclose their suicidal thoughts to someone. It is a huge and heavy burden to carry suicidal thoughts alone. Telling someone allows them to be heard, supported and helped.

It is so important to ask the question. In Chapter 7, I will explain more about the kind of direct questions you can ask to help someone to disclose their suicidal thoughts, and how you can assess someone's risk of suicide.

MYTH 5

"It's a selfish act."
Sadly, a depressed person is likely to think that they are a burden to their family and that they are being kind to their family by removing themselves from the world. This is how depression can distort the way someone is thinking. It can lead people to feel that they have no worth. It can mean that they no longer see themselves as they really are.

Describing it as "selfish" adds to the pain which they are feeling, and adds to the negative things they are probably already feeling about themselves in their depressed state, so it is really important to dispel this myth.

I have been supporting people in suicidal crisis for many years, and I know how often they think about and consider other people and worry about their loved ones. But they can reach a point where they descend deeper into crisis and lose sight of them, particularly if they go deeper into the "tunnel" of depression. Many of them are unwell at this point, or unable to think clearly and rationally anymore because their intense suffering or emotional distress is preventing rational thought.

MYTH 6

"It's weak to be suicidal."

In reality, a suicidal crisis can happen to people who have been extremely self-reliant throughout their life. During a family crisis, they may bury their own feelings and care for everyone else. They are often described as the rock of the family or "the strong one". Crucially, they may never learn to ask for help or support – and this is the key part. The pain of major life events can accumulate over the years. It stays buried inside because they never talk about it. Eventually, a final trigger may occur – one too many painful life events. This can "unlock" painful or traumatic events, which they have filed away in a compartment of their mind. The years of pain that have built up inside them may be released at this point. It can be overwhelming, and may trigger a suicidal crisis.

John, who I told you about in the last chapter, described this very powerfully. When his wife left him unexpectedly, he started to experience all the pain of previous losses, including the traumatic deaths of two family members which had happened many years ago. He said it was as if he had locked all this away in boxes in his head, but the shock of his wife leaving him "blew the lids off all the boxes".

MYTH 7

"It's attention-seeking."

This is suggesting that someone is telling people that they are feeling suicidal in order to get attention. It implies that they are trying to gain attention for negative reasons. It may also give the impression that we should not take what they are saying seriously.

You can frame this differently by saying: "They are drawing my attention to the fact that they are feeling suicidal." They are letting you know that they are in crisis and that they need help. It's important to always take this seriously.

I remember going out to see a young woman at her home and hearing a neighbour comment: "There's an ambulance outside her house every other week because she's harmed herself, or she says she's going to harm herself. Either that or the police are out looking for her because she is saying she is suicidal. It's just attention-seeking."

The neighbour did not know the reasons for the young woman's crises, though. The young woman was experiencing deep emotional pain. She was trying to cope with severe post-traumatic symptoms. We often find that people who have multiple crises have been through something very traumatic. This can be extremely destabilizing. Often, they have not yet had the right kind of help or treatment. They may not have had psychological therapy, either because it is too soon for them, or because there is some other reason why there is difficulty accessing it.

MYTH 8

"Only certain types of people become suicidal."

In reality, a suicidal crisis can happen to any one of us. It is usually a complex interplay of different factors which leads someone to feel suicidal. We all have a limit to what we can take before we become psychologically vulnerable. None of us is psychologically invincible.

It is so complex that it can be hard even for the person in crisis to see what has led to their own suicidal crisis. If they are asked, they may say that they don't know. We are complex beings, and our minds are complicated.

Sometimes it is only months or years after a suicidal crisis that someone can see all the different factors that may have led to it.

Depression can happen to any one of us. Depression can change and distort the way we think. It can make us vulnerable to a suicidal crisis.

When someone says that they cannot imagine ever becoming suicidal, I think it is that *they have not encountered the unique set of circumstances that might push them into a suicidal crisis.*

TALKING ABOUT "COMMITTING SUICIDE"

Up until 1961, suicide was considered a crime in the UK and in many other countries, and that is why people used the phrase "commit suicide" – because we talk about "committing" crimes. In 1961 the Suicide Act was passed in England, decriminalizing suicide.[9] Similarly, in the USA, individual states were starting to decriminalize suicide by the later 1960s. This means that the use of the word "commit" is no longer appropriate. It has negative associations, and links back to a time when there was less understanding of why someone develops suicidal thoughts.

Bereaved families who have lost a loved one to suicide can find the phrase particularly distressing, and this is a strong reason for considering the language that we use carefully. The phrase can contribute to the stigma around suicide.

As a result, we now use phrases like "died by suicide", or we say that someone "ended their life". Some people use the phrase "took their own life". It's important to understand that language is very individual, and it's about using language that an individual feels comfortable with.

Other recent changes in the law take us further away from criminal connotations. For example, in 2020 a judgement in the Supreme Court in the UK changed the standard of proof for suicide.[10] Before 2020, a coroner needed to be satisfied that a suicide had been proved "beyond reasonable doubt". That was the criminal standard of proof. Now, coroners use the civil standard of proof. It only needs to be proved "on the balance of probabilities" that someone died by suicide.

A further recent change in legal language is that coroners in the UK now talk about the "conclusion" to an inquest rather than the "verdict".

MYTH 9

"If someone is really determined to end their life, there is nothing that anyone can do about it."

If someone experiences a suicidal crisis, they may develop a strong intent to end their life at some point during the crisis. However, it is often a short-term feeling, because things have suddenly escalated. Sometimes this strong suicidal intent has been triggered by something that has just happened, which has felt overwhelming.

When someone experiences this very strong intent, it can feel like they have developed a kind of tunnel vision. All they can see is the goal of ending their life. It is as if everything they care about and everyone they love disappears into some far distant horizon. People who have experienced this often say that they could no longer hold their loved ones in their mind, at this point.

If we intervene to protect their life at this point, and they get the right help and support, it is likely that their suicidal intent will decrease as the hours and days pass.

EXPERIENCING SUICIDAL INTENT: MEGAN'S EXPERIENCE

Megan explained her experiences of suicidal intent. She had been having suicidal thoughts for several weeks. She had experienced a number of painful events recently, including the traumatic death of a family member. One day, she went to a bereavement support group meeting and learned that someone else she knew had died in very traumatic circumstances. This news came as a massive shock, at a time when she was very vulnerable. It was destabilizing and it caused a sudden escalation in her risk. She had strong thoughts of ending her life, which started very soon after the support group meeting ended. It very quickly turned into an immediate intention to end her life.

She finds it very hard now to understand how she suddenly felt so intent on ending her life at that point. She got on the bus to go home. She was barely aware of what was going on around her. She was experiencing the kind of "tunnel vision" I have described.

If I was to try to use a metaphor to help you understand it, I might say that it's like looking through a tube or telescope – all they can see at that point is their goal to end their life. This can prevent them from being aware of other people. In that moment, they may not be able to see them. They are usually disconnected from others – the other people are outside their field of vision. Megan explained: "It was as if they no longer existed – everyone I cared about had disappeared from my mind at that point."

Suddenly, someone on the bus started to speak to her. As the stranger continued to talk to her, it helped to disrupt the tunnel vision. The stranger helped to interrupt her focused suicidal intent. By speaking to her, she helped to make her aware of other people and her surroundings again. It was of course important that she got immediate professional help, and she called a crisis service when she arrived home.

Megan's experience shows how *connecting with the person who is at risk* is so important. Even when they have very focused intent, breaking through the barriers and connecting with them can make a difference.

Even when someone has a plan to end their life that continues over a period of days or weeks, they can absolutely be helped. They may carry out final acts as part of their preparations, as I will explain in Chapter 6 on warning signs. They may show other signs that make you suspect that they are planning to end their life, as that chapter also explains. If you suspect that they do have a plan, talking to them and asking about suicide (see Chapter 7) can be the start of disrupting their plans.

> This is the beginning of a period of time when your care and support, along with the essential intervention of professionals, can make such a difference.

Immediate professional help is vital, but the longer-term help, especially talking therapy (for example, psychological therapy) is so important, too. Once someone is out of immediate crisis, psychological therapy can help with the underlying reasons they wanted to end their life. In the UK, their doctor can make a referral for therapy under mental health services. I will explain how to access a psychologist in the USA and in other countries in Chapter 15.

MYTH 10

"Someone who dies by suicide will leave a note."
In reality, a high proportion of people who end their lives don't leave a note, because they are so highly distressed or so mentally unwell at that point that they are unable to do so.

Some people do leave a note, because it is important to them to leave an explanation, or because they want to leave practical instructions for arrangements after their death, such as funeral arrangements. In some cases, they may have written the note several days before ending their life as part of "final acts".

When there is no note, bereaved families who are desperately seeking to understand what may have led their loved one to end their life may be left with the question "why?" This can be a source of unbearable anguish and distress, as families try to find answers. Even when someone has left a note, it may be very short and may provide little information about what led them to end their life.

Talking to other people who have been bereaved by suicide, as well as to bereavement charities, can be part of the support which is so vital on this painful journey after the traumatic death of a loved one. I will focus again on bereavement by suicide in the next chapter.

IN SUMMARY

It's been important in this chapter to explain why the common myths and misinformation are incorrect, and to explain more about suicidal feelings and how and why they can occur. My aim throughout these early chapters is to increase your knowledge and understanding, in order to give you the best possible foundation for being able to help someone.

As well as affecting your ability to help someone, the myths have a far-reaching impact in our communities, making it harder for people to ask for help, and to be helped.

Additionally, some of these myths can be deeply distressing to people who have lost someone to suicide, adding to the emotional pain they are experiencing.

I hope that this chapter will help by creating wider understanding of suicidal feelings. We can all play a part in gently dispelling the myths when we hear them.

5

RISK FACTORS

In this chapter, you'll start to learn about assessing suicide risk. I'll explain some of the factors that can increase someone's risk of suicide, so that you can consider whether these risk factors apply to the person you are concerned about. If they *do* apply, I have included some of the things you can do to help them.

ASSESSING RISK

When we are assessing the suicide risk of our clients, we take into account many different factors, including:

- What they tell us explicitly (or implicitly) about suicidal thoughts or intention (if they tell us)
- Our knowledge and understanding of them as a person – what we know and have learned about them already
- Previous life events that may increase their risk
- Current life events that are causing distress, emotional pain or suffering
- Current circumstances that are impacting on their quality of life

- Other factors that make them vulnerable (such as not having supportive people around them in their personal life)
- Future known life events (for example, future events that they may be frightened about, or feel unable to cope with)
- Mental illness that may be impacting on their ability to think clearly
- Current high levels of emotional distress, which can affect their ability to think clearly
- Changes in their behaviour, which can signal increased risk
- Changes in their mood, which may lead to (or signal) increased risk
- Specific actions that raise our concerns (such as carrying out "final acts", which I'll talk about in the next chapter)
- Their body language/non-verbal cues

I'll explain more about these risk factors in this chapter and the chapters that follow.

RECOGNIZING THE RISK FACTORS

If you have known the person you are concerned about for a long time, you will probably have a good understanding of them. You will also probably have a good knowledge of past events in their life, and this can be really helpful when you are trying to assess their current risk of suicide. You will know if they have been through painful life events, which could be affecting them now.

And if you already know them well, and have a strong relationship with them, they are more likely to trust you and feel able to tell you about their suicidal thoughts. If you haven't known them for long, you can build trust with them by being caring and kind, showing your concern for them, giving your time, and being reliable and consistent. For example, if you say you are going to call them on a particular day/time or do something else for them, then do it – this is really important in allowing them to start to trust you.

> If someone finds it difficult to trust people, then they might have learned to trust people based on their actions rather than their words.

However long you have known someone, your previous knowledge of them means that you may notice other signs that can alert you to their increased risk, such as changes in their behaviour. For example, they may start to behave in a way that's different from usual or seems out of character. You are also more likely to notice if their mood changes. And crucially, your knowledge of them might allow you to notice small and subtle signs in their behaviour and demeanour, which can be signs of increased risk. Someone who knows them less well – such as a doctor meeting them for the first time – might be completely oblivious to these small signs. I'll talk about this more later on.

As I have explained before, it is rarely a single event that leads to a suicidal crisis. It is usually a combination of factors. However, there are a number of known factors that can increase someone's risk of suicide. In highlighting these known risk factors below, I would stress again that to assess risk accurately, we need to focus very much on the individual, and on the unique combination of factors that are increasing their risk of suicide.

Suicide Crisis' research into deaths by suicide in Gloucestershire in 2017-18 highlighted many of the following risk factors.

LOSS OF A LOVED ONE

During our research into deaths by suicide, we found that nearly half the individuals who took their own life had either *been bereaved or had experienced a breakup of a relationship* and it was documented that this had an impact on their suicide risk.

Bereavement

Most of us will know the aching loss and profound emotional pain of losing someone we love. Even if we knew that they were going to die, and we thought we were "emotionally prepared" for someone's death, the pain is usually vastly more intense and overwhelming than we could have ever imagined. Grief can involve many complicated feelings, too, including shock, guilt and anger. If someone has had a complicated relationship with the person who died, they can experience many different types of painful emotions.

For some of us, the grieving process becomes even more complex, perhaps because of the circumstances in which our loved one died. Professionals sometimes refer to "complicated grief". If the circumstances of the death were traumatic – for example if it was a sudden, unexpected or violent death – professionals talk about "traumatic grief". If they died in traumatic circumstances, it can be hard for us to start the grieving process. Whenever we think of them, we may find ourselves focusing on the way in which they died, rather than our memories of them. That can be so painful and distressing that we avoid thinking about them at all. This can disrupt the grieving process. It can stop us being able to grieve for them properly. This can have a very detrimental impact on someone's mental health because they are suppressing the painful emotions that are part of grief.

SEEKING HELP AFTER A TRAUMATIC BEREAVEMENT

After a traumatic bereavement, someone may also suffer post-traumatic symptoms (see later in this chapter). That's why trauma-focused therapy is usually so important – to help alleviate the post-traumatic symptoms, and help them process the traumatic aspect of the person's death, so that they can start to grieve. It's important to get professional help from a psychologist or counsellor, or from a bereavement charity. Counselling and therapy for traumatic grief can be accessed through psychiatric services and charities. Your care and support for your bereaved friend or loved one will make a significant difference, too. Keeping in contact with them, messaging or calling them, offering practical help, and small thoughtful acts of kindness all help. Just being there for them can mean so much.

Relationship break-up

A significant percentage of the people we see at our Suicide Crisis Centre have experienced a recent relationship break-up, and our research provided evidence of this risk factor, too. As well as experiencing emotional pain and feelings of acute loss, they can experience isolation and loneliness, and so by being there for them – supporting, caring and comforting them – you play an important role.

A MENTAL HEALTH CONDITION

This includes depression, post-traumatic stress disorder (and other trauma-related mental health conditions), eating disorders, anxiety disorders, bipolar disorder and schizophrenia and schizoaffective disorder.

It can be really helpful to learn more about the diagnosis that your friend or family member has been given – by reading books or contacting the national or local charity for the particular mental health condition. Often, better understanding means you can help more. Clients at our Suicide Crisis Centres have sometimes told us that they wished their loved ones understood more about *how their mental health condition affects them, and the challenges they face.*

DRUG OR ALCOHOL USE

In our research into deaths by suicide, we found that 60 per cent of the people who died by suicide were using drugs or alcohol in the months leading up to their death. In most cases, it was apparent that they were using drugs or alcohol to try to suppress painful feelings or distressing memories, often caused by traumatic events.

ISOLATION

Living alone can be a risk factor, especially if there is a lack of emotional support from family or friends. If someone does not have meaningful relationships and has little contact with other people, they can be at increased risk. In these circumstances, your connection with them can be a very important part of alleviating their isolation. Research published in 2020 suggests that men who live alone are particularly vulnerable.[11]

PREVIOUS SUICIDE ATTEMPTS

When someone has already made a suicide attempt, it is more likely that they will make another attempt. But it is not inevitable.

It is so important that they receive intensive professional support in the days and weeks afterwards. Many people will have sustained physical damage, either external or internal – or indeed both. This can be temporary or permanent damage.

The body is often in internal chaos after a suicide attempt, particularly after an overdose. The toxins can affect the body for many days afterwards, or even longer. This is in addition to the mental and psychological distress that they were feeling at the time of the attempt, which they can still be experiencing. This combination of physical and mental turmoil makes them even more vulnerable: there is a real risk that they will make a further suicide attempt, and that is why intensive support by mental health professionals or crisis services is so vital.

A FAMILY HISTORY OF SUICIDE

When someone dies by suicide, it is a deeply traumatic event, which causes unimaginable pain and suffering to the people closest to them. By giving your support to their family member, friend or work colleague, you can help so much. Letting them know that you care, and that you are there for them, giving your time, listening, keeping in contact and messaging – all of this is so helpful.

SUPPORT FOR PEOPLE WHO HAVE BEEN BEREAVED BY SUICIDE

Earlier in this chapter I mentioned traumatic grief, and how the grieving process can be more complex, and how someone may also experience post-traumatic symptoms as a result. A death by suicide is particularly traumatic. As well as the specialist psychological help I described, there are national charities that provide support for people who have been bereaved by suicide. They are often set up by people who have themselves been bereaved by suicide. I have given details of how to contact them at the end of this book.

If someone in the family has died by suicide, there is an increased risk that another family member may take their own life. There can also be an increased risk of suicide for other people who knew the person.

A report by the Royal College of Psychiatrists in 2020 highlighted the wide range of people who are impacted by a suicide bereavement, including relatives, friends, partners and the professionals (including psychiatrists) who cared for the person before their death.[12]

A research paper in 2016 showed that bereavement by suicide "is a specific factor for suicide attempt among young bereaved adults, whether they are related to the deceased or not". So the death by suicide of *friends or non-blood relatives* creates a significant risk, too.[13]

TRAUMATIC EVENTS

Traumatic events include events that can trigger fear, shock, horror and helplessness. Examples of traumatic events include violent physical assaults, domestic violence, witnessing a violent or traumatic death, war, natural disasters, man-made disasters and serious accidents.

Traumatic events can be extremely destabilizing. However, if someone is well supported by family or friends in the weeks after the event, it can be extremely helpful to their eventual recovery.

As well as running suicide crisis centres, the charity runs a separate Trauma Centre. This is because we know how important it is that people are well supported after trauma – to prevent them from deteriorating and experiencing a suicidal crisis.

Someone who has been through a traumatic event may go on to develop symptoms of post-traumatic stress disorder. These can include:

- Re-living: You may have flashbacks, where you feel that you are re-living the event again. You may have repeated nightmares or intrusive thoughts about the incident.
- Avoiding: You may avoid people or places that remind you of the incident. You may also avoid thinking about the event.
- Being on high alert: This is known as "hypervigilance". It is as if you are expecting more dangerous or frightening things to happen and so you are "on your guard" all the time. It may mean that you are easily startled: you may jump when you hear a noise, when other people don't seem to notice it.

Support immediately after traumatic events (from family and friends) can make a significant difference to someone's recovery.

SELF-HARM

Self-harm is about someone intentionally harming themselves. It may not be life-threatening harm. *If someone self-harms, they may not be trying to end their life.* The reasons why someone self-harms can be complex. Self-harm can be about releasing painful emotions, which feel unbearable. This can help someone to feel able to stay alive in the short term. It can be a way in which they try to manage their distress.

There are other reasons why someone may self-harm. It can be about trying to take control when they are feeling powerless. For some people, it is about trying to punish themselves if they have negative feelings toward themselves.

Even though the self-harm may not be an attempt to end their life, research has shown that if someone has a history of self-harm, there is an increased risk that they will end their life by suicide at some point.[12]

The report by the Royal College of Psychiatrists in 2020 refers to recent research which shows that almost half of people who die by suicide "have previously harmed themselves". The report stresses how important it is that staff carry out a thorough mental health assessment when someone comes to a hospital

Emergency Department after self-harming – and that they react with understanding and compassion. Safety plans and follow-up by professionals are also highlighted as important in the report.

PHYSICAL ILL HEALTH

In our research into deaths by suicide, we noted that 36 per cent of the individuals who had died had significant health issues, which impacted upon their suicide risk.

We know that chronic pain can be a particular risk factor. Many of our clients have found that a referral to a specialist pain clinic at the local hospital gave them access to treatments for chronic pain that were not available from their doctor in the community.

ARGUMENTS AND CONFLICT

In our research, we found that 20 per cent of the individuals who ended their life were involved in an argument in the hours before they died, often immediately before their death. In Chapter 14, I'll explain more about anger and suicide risk, and how you can help.

POVERTY OR FINANCIAL PROBLEMS AND DEBT

During our research, we found that 20 per cent of the people who died by suicide had money problems or debt problems, which had a significant impact on them. A report, Dying from Inequality, published by the Samaritans in 2017 explained how financial instability, debt and poverty can increase suicide risk.[14]

BEING IN THE CRIMINAL JUSTICE SYSTEM

There are increased risks at every stage in the criminal justice system, whether someone is being investigated by the police in connection with a criminal offence, or is in prison having been convicted.

According to our research, 16 per cent of the individuals who died by suicide *were under criminal investigation at the time of death*, and this had a significant impact upon their risk. In some cases, it seemed to be the factor impacting most upon their risk of suicide. The fear of the outcome of the investigation (prison, and in some cases a fear of other consequences of conviction such as publicity and loss of reputation) had a major effect.

There can be further increased risk when someone goes to prison. The Howard League for Penal Reform published a report in 2016, Preventing Prison Suicide, which showed that the number of prisoners who took their own lives had increased substantially since 2011.[15] They found that by 2016, a prisoner was dying by suicide every three days in England and Wales. The figures published in 2019 were similar to those from 2016.

The report highlights the fact that there are now fewer staff in prisons, and this makes it harder for prisoners to build relationships with staff, which could have been supportive. Staff shortages can also mean prisoners spend more time isolated in their cells. Contact from friends and family by letter (and phone/visits where possible) becomes even more important.

LOSS OF CONTACT WITH YOUR CHILDREN

If someone is unable to see their children, it is of course profoundly distressing and painful. This may happen when a relationship ends and a partner moves away, taking the children with them. Or an individual may lose custody of their children in the family court after a divorce or separation. It becomes much harder if contact is restricted or prevented, either by the courts or social services, or if an ex-partner refuses to let them see their children.

At our Suicide Crisis Centres, we see so much evidence of the impact on parents of being unable to see their children. Many parents had their contact restricted because of their mental health problems during a particularly difficult time. When they become well again, they may have to go through a court procedure to have greater access to their children.

Our research showed that losing access to one's children was a significant risk factor in death by suicide.

OTHER LIFE EVENTS (INVOLVING LOSS OR CHANGE)

Significant life events that trigger *loss or change* can have an impact on suicide risk. These include losing a job and starting university.

Losing a job is extremely painful for most of us. For some people, their sense of identity and self-esteem is strongly linked to their ability to do their job. If they lose their job, they may feel they have lost that part of their identity. Their self-esteem may plummet. It may feel as though they have lost their role in life. Work can also give us a strong sense of purpose – we are contributing and making a difference. Additionally, a job usually gives people daily contact with work colleagues. So there is the loss of social contact and supportive work relationships, too. If they have worked together for many years, this can be a particularly painful loss.

Later in the book I will explain why it is so important to help people recognize their innate worth, which is separate from the job that they do. I will explain how you can help them to see that who they are is so much more important than what they do.

Many people find voluntary work provides a way to contribute in a very meaningful way, while they consider what they might want to do next.

Other major life changes include starting university or college. Prior to going to university or college, many students have been living at home with family, or near friends who they have known for years. Starting university can feel a lonely experience for some people – and it can feel a sudden transition to independence. They may be at a university or college on the other side of the country from their home, living alone or with a group of students who they don't really know.

The course itself may seem daunting and challenging. They may be struggling with aspects of the course or may feel hugely under pressure to meet coursework deadlines. They may feel under pressure to achieve.

Some students have taken on a job to finance their degree and they may quickly find that the combination of a job and full-time academic study creates huge stresses, as well as physical and mental exhaustion.

Counselling services are available on most university or college campuses, as well as other student support services. Regular phone calls, messages and visits from friends and family from their home town can be extremely supportive, too.

Some universities in the UK are introducing opt-in schemes that allow the university to contact parents if students are experiencing mental health difficulties. It was the father of a student who died by suicide who asked for the scheme to be introduced. In its first year of operation at Bristol University, 94 per cent of students opted into the scheme.

In the USA, the Jed Foundation is a non-profit organization which assists schools and colleges to develop effective campus-wide strategies to protect students' mental health and to prevent suicide.

A CHANGE IN CARE OR CARE SETTING

There are increased risks around the time of *a change in care or care setting*. A significant change of care includes a new psychiatric care team becoming involved in a patient's care (for example, a change of care coordinator and psychiatrist) or a move from psychiatric hospital to community care.

BULLYING AND VICTIMIZATION

Bullying can have such a devastating impact on someone's self worth. It can be frightening, isolating and can leave someone feeling utterly powerless. It can lead to feelings of rejection and exclusion. It can take place in the community, in the workplace and in schools, colleges and universities.

It is so important to get help and advice from anti-bullying charities, and to access counselling and support. Charities in the UK which provide helplines include Bullying UK. In the USA there is Stomp Out Bullying, and Bully Zero in Australia. Contact details are at the end of the book.

A FEELING OF NOT FITTING IN OR NOT BELONGING

Feeling that you don't fit in can be very hard. It can happen as a result of being excluded by other people, or being made to feel that you are different in some way – and that this "difference" is negative, rather than positive. It is of course this "difference" that often becomes our greatest contribution – something we bring to the world that no one else can.

Many of us eventually become very comfortable about what makes us different, but it can be hard, particularly when we are younger. There is often much more pressure to fit in and to be the same as our peer group in school and college, and in our early adult life.

AUTISM

Autism affects how people communicate and interact with the world – and it affects individuals in different ways.

In the Māori language of New Zealand, "*takiwātanga*" is the word for autism and it means "in their own time and space" – a beautiful phrase. It seems to highlight the fact that we should adapt to the individual pace and timing of someone who has autism, rather than expect that they should adapt to ours.

In looking at reasons why someone with autism may be at increased risk of suicide, we know that our clients who have autism often cite social isolation and loneliness as contributory factors. They may also experience bullying. And they may find it harder to identify or communicate how they are feeling, and so if they are experiencing distress or emotional pain, it can be harder to seek help or get help. It's important that services adapt to meet the needs of individuals. For example, someone who has autism may feel uncomfortable with phone services, preferring to text and email.

You can help by explaining (to any relevant services) some of the specific changes that would make things easier for your friend or family member, such as the way in which they communicate with them.

For additional help and support, there is the National Autistic Society in the UK, the Autism Society in the USA and Autism Awareness in Australia. Their contact details are at the end of this book.

LESBIAN, GAY, BISEXUAL AND TRANSGENDER PEOPLE

People in the LGBTQ+ community can be at greater risk of suicide, particularly if they are experiencing discrimination or verbal harassment, abuse or violence as a result of their sexual identity. Other factors which can increase risk include: if there is a lack of support from family and friends, conflict with family about their sexual identity, rejection by family, or a lack of respect or recognition of their gender identity. Research in the USA found that LGBT students in grades 9 to 12 were three times more likely than heterosexual students to have seriously considered attempting suicide.[16]

Also in the USA, 40 per cent of transgender people who responded to a national survey said that they had attempted suicide in their lifetime. Almost all of them had attempted suicide before the age of 25 (96 per cent).[17]

In the same USA national survey, 13 per cent of young people who reported high levels of support from family, friends or one special person reported attempting suicide in the past year, compared with 22 per cent of those with lower levels of support.

In the UK, the national charity LGBT Foundation provides a helpline for anyone who is struggling with their mental health. In the USA, the Trevor Project provides crisis intervention, suicide prevention services and a national helpline, and Australia has the Q Life Counselling Service. Their contact details are at the end of this book.

DIFFICULTY IN ACCESSING MENTAL HEALTH SERVICES

We know that it can sometimes be difficult to access mental health services. There are limited resources and staff shortages. There are other reasons why it can be hard to access mental health services. There may be waiting lists for specialist treatment such as psychological therapies.

Statistics in the UK show that around a third of the people who die by suicide are under mental health services (or had recently been).[18] However, in our research we found evidence that many of the people who took their life had been trying to access mental health services in the days or weeks before they died – or their family or friends had been contacting psychiatric services to try to get them urgent help.

We found that if we factored in the people who were trying (unsuccessfully) to access psychiatric services shortly before they died, the number would be much higher than a third. If they had successfully accessed mental health services, then 60 per cent would have been receiving their care. *If they had been able to access this vital care, there is a possibility that they might have survived.*

If your friend or family member is struggling to get the right longer-term mental health care, there are some suggestions that may help in Chapter 15.

PREMENSTRUAL DYSPHORIC DISORDER (PMDD)

PMDD is a severe form of premenstrual syndrome which affects mood and emotions, and also causes physical symptoms, in the week or two before someone's period. It can also cause some people to experience severe depression or anxiety, and some people experience suicidal thoughts.

If your friend or family member is experiencing PMDD, there are treatments available, and their doctor or physician can give advice and make referrals. You can help by learning and understanding more about PMDD and asking your friend/family member how it affects them personally. The International Association for Premenstrual Disorders can provide support (including peer support) and information.

IN SUMMARY

If the person you are concerned about has some of the risk factors in this chapter, it does not mean that they will end their life. But being aware of their individual risk factors can help you to understand and support them even more. And it means that you can assist them in getting very specific types of help, some of which are mentioned in this chapter.

WARNING SIGNS

In this chapter, I'll talk about some of the warning signs that indicate that someone may be having suicidal thoughts. I'll explain the kind of changes you might see in their behaviour, their mood or in the kind of things that they say.

Some of these changes can be an indication that they are planning to end their life, or even that there is an immediate risk of suicide. I will explain how to respond and what kind of help you can get for them.

The warning signs for each individual can be very different and unique to them, however. Some people won't say anything but may give non-verbal signs through their body language or voice tone, and I'll explain more about that in Chapter 9, Beyond Words.

WHAT THEY MAY SAY

In each of these situations, it's important to involve a doctor, crisis service or mental health professional that same day.

Talking about wanting to die or about killing themselves

Your friend or loved one may make direct comments about wanting to end their life. They may be very explicit. However, some people may say it in quite a casual way (as I explained in Chapter 4).

A remark like "I don't know why I don't just kill myself", or "I might as well kill myself", should always be taken seriously.

It is sometimes easier for the person at risk to introduce the subject in a casual way, because suicide can be so difficult to talk about. It's so important to get help from a doctor or crisis service on the same day. In our research into deaths by suicide, we found that some people made these kinds of remarks casually in the days and weeks before ending their life.

Talking about feeling a loss of hope, that things can never improve, or that there is no reason to live

When someone is deeply depressed, they may feel that there is no hope for the future. Sometimes our clients talk about feeling as though they are in the middle of a dark tunnel, which appears to have no end. The tunnel *does* of course have an end, and light at the end of it; they may not be able to see it in the midst of their depression, though.

Talking negatively about themselves

They may say: "I'm nothing", "I feel I have nothing to offer", or they may say that they are worthless. It can be heartbreaking to hear this. One of my current clients – a caring, giving man who has supported other people throughout his life – tells me that he is "useless" and "wasting people's time". It is in this way that depression is influencing his thinking.

In Chapter 11, I will explain how you can help someone who is thinking in this way.

Saying that they are a burden, or that people would be better off without them

Depression can make someone feel that they are a burden to other people – to their family, friends and to professionals who are supporting them. They may start to feel that it would be better for their loved ones if they were not here. In reality, of course, their loved ones would be devastated if they were not here.

Talking about feelings of guilt

This can include guilt about family or friends supporting them emotionally or financially. It can be linked to the feeling of being a burden. They may also express guilt about services needing to support them.

They may also talk about feeling guilty about things they have done – this may include things they did many years ago. When someone is depressed, they can focus on painful events from their past, and may focus on what they feel they did wrongly, or what they didn't do at the time.

Talking about feeling unbearable pain

They may talk about feeling unbearable emotional pain. Their suffering may have reached a point where it feels that they cannot stand it any longer. Your emotional support can make a difference, as I will explain later. But get professional help for them on that same day. Thoughts of suicide can be about wanting an end to the pain, rather than actually wanting to die.

Saying that they feel trapped in a situation

They may say things like: "I can't see any way out of this." Ending their life may start to feel like a way of escaping from a situation in which they feel trapped.

BEHAVIOUR: WHAT THEY MAY DO

All the changes of behaviour I am about to describe are a cause for immediate concern because they can indicate an escalation in the person's suicide risk, and some of them can indicate that someone is planning to end their life imminently. Support them by assisting them to get help from a doctor, mental health service or crisis service that same day.

Reckless or dangerous behaviour

This can include driving too fast or behaving in a way that puts them at risk of harm. They may show no concern about the consequences to themselves.

Sudden outbursts of rage or aggression, or violence toward property

At our Suicide Crisis Centre, we are always very concerned when one of our clients suddenly starts to express rage or tells us that they found themselves smashing up crockery, cups or other items. They may also start swearing and using language that they would not usually use. They often say how out of character it is. It is a warning sign that things are escalating. They are less able to control their emotions and as a result, they may have less control over what they do next.

Becoming more withdrawn and quiet

Sometimes it is the opposite – someone will become quiet and they may retreat into themselves.

Isolating themselves by withdrawing from friends, family and the wider community

Someone who is usually willing to have social contact may suddenly withdraw from everyone they know.

No longer participating in activities that were important to them

They may stop doing things that usually matter very much to them, including hobbies or sport or creative activities.

Putting affairs in order

When someone is planning to end their life, they may carry out "final acts" or put their affairs in order. For example, they might visit a solicitor to arrange to write a will, or they start to put their business affairs in order. They may do this to make it easier for their colleagues to take over from them after their death. They may make financial arrangements to make sure their family is secure. They may make other arrangements for people or animals they care about – giving up their pets or arranging for them to be cared for by someone else, for example.

If you know or suspect that they are carrying out some of these actions, try to talk to them, to share your concerns with them. Ask the questions about suicidal thoughts that are in the next chapter. Offer your support and help. It is also vital to make urgent contact with a doctor or crisis service.

If your friend or loved one is not willing to talk to professionals and/or they tell you that there is nothing to worry about and you nevertheless remain concerned, call a crisis service or doctor to ask for advice. At our Suicide Crisis Centre, we are always very willing to give advice about what to do, and many other crisis services will do the same.

Saying goodbye to other people

It may not be obvious that they are saying goodbye. They may visit unexpectedly, or visit family members who they have not seen for a very long time. Try to gently explore the reasons for the unexpected visit. You might say to them: "It is really wonderful to see you but I am concerned about why you might be visiting me at this time." Or if they have visited another family member, ask how the visit went, and express the same concern about the timing of the visit. Then lead onto the questions in the next chapter to try to find out if they are having suicidal thoughts.

Saying sorry

They may unexpectedly say that they are sorry. It may be unclear what they are apologizing for – they may be unspecific about this. Sometimes clients will send us a message that simply says "I am sorry", when they have no apparent reason to apologize to us. This unexpected apology (with no further explanation) can sometimes mean: "I am sorry for what I am going to do", or "I am sorry, I cannot stay alive anymore and I am going to end my life."

Bereaved parents have also sometimes told us that their loved one apologized unexpectedly to them shortly before they took their own life. It was not clear to them why they were apologizing. One parent told us that she had assumed that her son was saying sorry for being in crisis, but she later believed that it was a sign that he was already planning to end his life.

The apology might be spoken or in a text, letter or email. You can respond by saying: "Thank you so much for your message. I want to reassure you that you have absolutely no need to apologize." Then you can try to explore why they were apologizing. You can go on to say: "Can we talk about this?" and "Can I ask how you are feeling at this time?" and then lead on to the questions about suicidal thoughts in the next chapter.

Saying thank you

Similarly, they might say thank you, when it is not clear what they are thanking you for.

They might be more specific: if they are preparing to end their life, they might thank people for everything they have done to support and help them.

One of our clients took a dear friend out to lunch "as a thank you for all your support". Our client was still in a period of suicidal crisis, and their friend realized that this might be a warning sign that he was planning to end his life, just as we did.

You can say to them: "I'm concerned about you. I'm concerned about why you might be thanking me at this time", and then lead up to the questions about suicidal thoughts in the next chapter.

Giving away treasured possessions

They may give away things that mean a lot to them – perhaps to friends or loved ones. They may put their much-loved pet in someone else's care, when they have plans to end their life. Again, this is a time to express your concern, explore why they might be giving things away (which are precious to them) at this time, and lead up to the questions in the next chapter.

Posting on social media

Some people will make explicit statements on social media about wanting to die. But often the warning signs are less obvious. You may notice a change in their posts – signs that they appear low in mood or that things are difficult.

Sometimes people share songs on social media that describe emotional pain and distress. The songs may be about losing someone they love, or about feeling alone. The words of the songs can express how they feel. They may be trying to convey this. It may be too hard to actually say how they are feeling, but the song does it for them.

It can be very helpful to start a dialogue with them via private message on social media. For example, you could write something like: "I was listening to the song you shared and I just wanted to check how you are feeling?" This can be enough to open the communication.

Researching suicide methods

Looking for information about how to end their life, including searching online, is one of the most obvious warning signs. Sometimes our clients tell us that they have been doing this. Friends or family members may tell you. When someone is planning suicide, it can sometimes be extremely hard for them to hold that information inside them. Sometimes they desperately want to tell someone, so that they are not carrying the enormous burden of their suicide plan alone. It can feel so unbearably hard to be on that journey alone.

CHANGES IN MOOD

Some of these changes could be a sign of an immediate risk of a suicide attempt so it's time to contact a doctor, a crisis service or a mental health clinician who can speak to them that same day.

Becoming more depressed

You may notice that their depression has become much deeper over a period of days.

Becoming much more anxious

Their anxiety levels are so high that it feels like there is no respite from it. They may say that they never have any peace from it – that their mind is never allowed to rest.

Agitation

They may be agitated and restless. They might pace up and down, wring their hands or make other repetitive movements that indicate distress.

Becoming suddenly calm

They may suddenly become calm after a period of anxiety or depression. This may be because they are feeling a sense of relief or a sense of peace because of the awareness that their life will soon be over. It can be a sign that they have made a decision to end their life.

A brighter mood after a period of depression

A sudden lift in mood after a period of depression could be a sign that the person has made a decision to end their life.

As part of our research into deaths by suicide, we attended inquests. We noted that doctors or family members often commented that the person had seemed brighter in mood shortly before their death.

There are reasons why this can indicate increased risk:

1. When the person's mood starts to improve a little, they may gain the energy needed to end their life, which was lacking while deeply depressed.
2. Some people may appear bright (or even elated) once they have made a decision to end their life.

It is understandable that we may feel relief when someone's mood seems to lift. However, it is still a time to be cautious and watchful, and a time to ask questions about risk. And it is a time to ask for advice from professionals – particularly from a crisis service or mental health service – they will recognize this as a possible warning sign.

THE APPARENT ABSENCE OF WARNING SIGNS

We sometimes hear people say: "There were no warning signs", and I will explain in Chapter 9 how it is possible for some people to mask their suicide risk or indeed to intentionally cover up their suicidal feelings – often to try to protect other people from the pain and distress of knowing they are at risk of suicide. Of course, family and friends would want to know, and have the chance to help.

IN SUMMARY

It can feel very frightening if you notice warning signs, so as well as getting help for the person at risk, it's important to have support for yourself, and to be able to talk through your own feelings and fears with someone, whether it's a friend, family member, a helpline or a professional.

If you have noticed any of the warning signs in this chapter, or any other signs that make you concerned that someone may be thinking of ending their life or is at risk of suicide, the next chapter explains how to ask specific and direct questions about suicidal thoughts, and suicidal intent.

PART 2

HOW TO HELP

7

ASKING ABOUT SUICIDAL THOUGHTS

These are the important questions to ask when you are trying to find out:

- **If someone is having suicidal thoughts,** and
- **How immediate their risk of suicide is**

These have to be direct questions because you are trying to get a very clear idea of their risk.

Research shows that asking direct questions about suicide helps to protect someone's life, and that it does *not* put the idea into their head.

It's understandable that you might feel very apprehensive about asking the question. You may be fearful of their answer; afraid to know that someone you love is having thoughts of ending their life. It is what we dread hearing. Or you might be worried about how they will react. But in asking the question, and allowing them to tell you, you are opening the door to help and support. *You are significantly increasing their chance of surviving.* It can be so hard for them to disclose thoughts of ending their life. Your questions are an invitation to tell you. For many people, it will be such a relief to be able to disclose it to someone.

You may also feel worried about what to do if you find out that your friend, colleague or loved one is at risk of suicide. You may worry about the sudden responsibility of knowing this. If they are at immediate risk of suicide, it will be important to involve a crisis service, doctor or medical professional straight away. You will not be on your own in this situation. You will be able to link your friend or loved one to the right help.

HOW TO START

It often helps to explain the context: why you are asking the questions. You can lead up to the direct questions about suicide risk, by first of all exploring how things are with them. You can start by explaining that you are concerned about them – perhaps because you have noticed a change in their mood or behaviour, or just because you have a gut feeling that something is wrong. "I've noticed that you seem low in mood lately. I've been concerned about you. I wondered if there is anything I can do to help." "I've noticed that we haven't seen you at the club recently. We've missed you and I wondered how things are going for you."

Their response may help you to find out about any recent events that might be risk factors, or may help to explain the change in mood or behaviour.

They may be very willing to talk to you. It may allow them to release many of the very difficult and painful emotions that have been building up inside them. Or they may say very little. They may try to "close down" the conversation by giving short answers such as "I'm okay", or "everything's fine", but their body language and voice tone may suggest otherwise. They might avoid looking at you or their gaze might be fixed on the floor. Their body language may be very closed (crossed arms and legs).

If they *do* try to close down the conversation, you can gently persist by saying something like: "I am still concerned. I know that sometimes, when life becomes really difficult and painful, a person may start to have suicidal thoughts." This leads on to the first direct question about suicide:

1. "Are you having suicidal thoughts?" or "Have you been having thoughts of ending your life?"

If they say yes, it can help to gently ask for more information (if you haven't already explored it in the lead-up to the question about suicidal thoughts).

You can ask: "Can you tell me what's led to this?" As I said before, some people will welcome this opportunity to talk about what events have led them to this point. But some people may not feel able to talk about things yet. They may be too exhausted, or fearful. They may not have the words yet. It may be too painful or distressing to talk about it. They may be so used to putting up a front that they don't know how to respond. Sometimes they may not be sure what has led them to feel that they want to end their life. If they are very depressed, for example, there may not be any actual events they can pinpoint as having led them to such a dark place.

If they tell you that they have been through something very traumatic, it's important not to try to draw out detailed information about the event from them. It can be very harrowing for them to "re-live" the event. A psychologist or other appropriate professional will know how to do this safely, so it's important to leave this delicate work to them.

Next, you need to find out whether they have started to make *plans* or *preparations* to end their life:

2a. "Have you thought about how you would do it?"

It's important to find out if they have gone a stage further in their suicidal thinking – thinking about a suicide method. If they are thinking about a particular suicide method or they have decided on a suicide method, their risk is greater.

There is a difference between "Yes, I have been thinking about... (and they name a suicide method)" and "Yes, I am going to... (and they name their suicide method)."

We need to be very concerned about both answers, because they both mean that the person is at greater risk. But the person who says they are "going to..." is at immediate risk.

It is the difference between *thinking about* something and *planning or intending* to do something.

If they have told you, "Yes, I have been *thinking about* (a particular suicide method)", then explore this further. Check whether they also have a plan. They may not give you all the information you need in their answer to this question. You can ask:

2b. "Do you have a plan to end your life?" or "Are you planning to end your life?"

If they say yes, try to find out as much information as possible about their plan.

Ask them: "Can you tell me about the plan?"

If they say no: if they are having suicidal thoughts but they tell you that they have not gone any further in their plans or preparations, it is still important to involve a doctor or crisis service. Professionals will play an important role in helping to prevent them from deteriorating and going deeper into suicidal crisis.

You can say something like: "I really want to help and support you as much as I can while you are having suicidal thoughts. It's also important that we talk to a professional to make sure that you have the best possible help."

3. "Have you got your suicide method already?"

If they say yes to Question 2, it's important to find out if they have already acquired what they need to carry out their chosen suicide method.

Ask: "Have you got what you need to end your life already?" or "Have you got your suicide method already?"

Or, if they talk generally about going to a type of place to end their life, it's important to try to find out whether they have chosen a specific location.

If they *have* already acquired their chosen suicide method, or they *have* decided on a specific location, the risk is even greater.

Now you need to ask about timeframe – to find out how immediate the risk is:

4. "Have you thought about when you would do it?" or "Have you planned when you are going to do it?"

If they tell you that they are planning to end their life today, or very soon, then it's important to involve other services as quickly as you can. Stay with them in the meantime, if you possibly can, while you wait for help to arrive. You can call emergency services if there is an immediate risk to life.

Ambulance crews are very used to responding to people who are at immediate risk of suicide. A mental health emergency is as urgent as a physical health emergency.

You can take them to the Emergency Department at the local hospital yourself, or you can contact a crisis service or on-call doctor at the doctor's surgery.

Next, you need to check whether they have already tried to end their life.

5. "Have you already tried to end your life today, or in the last few days?"

Ask whether they have already attempted suicide – they may have swallowed something harmful earlier in the day, for example, which places their life at immediate risk.

A drug overdose taken several days earlier may still carry a risk of death or serious harm several days later, so it's important to get medical help.

6. "Have you ever attempted suicide in the past?"

Ask about past suicide attempts, too.

> If someone has attempted suicide before at any point in their life, this increases their risk.

If they have not attempted to use their suicide method yet, explain that you would like to remove any items from their home which they could use to end their life. These would be items that are related to their chosen method of suicide. Explain that you want to keep your friend or loved one safe by doing this. They may be willing for you to take the items, but if not, then tell the emergency services, or their doctor or crisis service. It will be important for them to know that the person at risk still has what they need to end their life at home.

FEARS AROUND GETTING HELP

When you tell your friend, colleague or family member that you want to make sure that they get the right help, they may feel apprehensive. They may be worried about what will happen next. You can reassure them that the professionals will want to help. They may say that they are worried that they will be "sectioned" (detained under a section of the Mental Health Act in the UK)[19] which means being admitted involuntarily to a psychiatric hospital.

But most people who have suicidal thoughts – or even a plan to end their life – don't get detained or admitted to psychiatric hospital against their will. In the UK, they will usually be offered help in the community instead. This can involve regular – often daily – visits from the mental health crisis team. Their role is to provide support and strategies to help someone to survive their crisis. The crisis teams (sometimes called "crisis resolution and home treatment teams") were set up as an alternative to psychiatric hospital. *Doctors usually only consider sectioning someone after they have tried all other options first.*

In most countries, it is possible to have a voluntary admission, which means someone chooses to go into psychiatric hospital for a period of time. Some people want to be in hospital – they feel they will be safer and will receive therapeutic support there.

They may feel more reassured if you go with them to the doctor's surgery or crisis service. You will be providing support and encouragement. Also, it can be hard for them to tell a professional what they have told you. They may welcome your help in telling the professional that they are having suicidal thoughts.

A NOTE ABOUT HOW RISK CAN CHANGE

When you ask about suicidal thoughts, your friend or family member may tell you that they have been having thoughts of suicide, but they may also say: "I don't think I would actually do it", or "I would never actually do it." They may go on to explain that there are reasons why they would not end their life.

This is reassuring to hear, but we know that things can change in the days and weeks afterwards. They may become more depressed, for example, and depression can change the way they think. They may lose sight of the things that are keeping them alive right now. This is why it's so important that they are helped and supported at an early stage. It's still vital to involve their doctor or a crisis service.

Sadly, I have spoken to parents and attended inquests (as part of our research into deaths by suicide) where they have explained that their loved one told them that they were having suicidal thoughts, but that they would never actually end their life (and they gave reasons why not). A few weeks later that changed, and tragically they ended their life.

8

UNDERSTANDING, EMPATHIZING AND CONNECTING

In the previous chapter, we focused on asking the right questions to find out if your friend or family member is having suicidal thoughts, or if they have a plan to end their life.

When your friend or loved one tells you that they are feeling suicidal, it will be important to them that they feel that *you understand their risk of suicide – that you have taken it seriously.*

By involving professionals (such as a crisis service, doctor or emergency services) you are showing them that you have understood the risk. You can say: "I am really concerned about you, and it's important that I contact a crisis service/doctor/emergency services to make sure that you get the right help."

THE IMPACT OF YOUR REACTIONS

It can be so painful to find out that your friend or loved one is having suicidal thoughts. As I explained in Chapter 1, this can cause some people to "block it out". They may be unable to absorb or accept the reality that the person is in crisis. It is as if they are thinking: "This can't be happening." This can lead them to try to normalize the situation and say things like: "Oh, you'll be all right."

This initial sense of denial is understandable, but it is likely to leave the person in crisis feeling that their suicide risk has not been recognized: "They can't see that I am at risk of suicide. They have not heard me."

WHAT IS IMPORTANT

They want to feel safe and secure in your support, and an important part of this is feeling that you *understand their risk of suicide.*

It will continue to be important to them that they feel heard at every stage, as you support them in the days and weeks that follow – that you are not dismissing what they are saying and feeling, and that you are trying to understand.

> As you continue to support your friend, colleague or loved one, it can be very helpful to use the kind of "active listening skills" that counsellors learn about at the beginning of their training.

Don't worry if you find it hard to remember all the active listening skills in this chapter, especially if you are starting to support someone for the first time. If you only remember one or two things, that's still really helpful. And if you can remember to "reflect the other person's emotions", that is one of the most helpful things you can do for your friend or loved one. I'll explain about that later in this chapter.

ACTIVE LISTENING

While you are listening, you are not just passively receiving what the other person tells you. You are communicating something to them all the time, even if it is not with your words.

You can communicate your care and concern – and the fact that you are listening attentively – in many different ways. It is not just communicated through what you say. Your body language also helps to convey it.

The following are some ways that you can demonstrate active listening.

Your body language

Open posture: An open posture (arms uncrossed and relaxed) gives out the message that you are open and receptive to hearing what someone is saying. An example of a closed posture is having your arms crossed in front of your body, and your legs crossed. This can look defensive, almost as if you have created a symbolic physical barrier that is keeping the other person out.

Eye contact: It's natural to look away sometimes, but eye contact shows that you are focused and attentive.

Nodding: It can be helpful to nod gently and briefly at appropriate times, as they talk. This provides encouragement to them, and shows that you are being supportive. It can help to reassure them that you are listening attentively, too. Two or three gentle nods from time to time work well, rather than vigorous and prolonged nodding, which may distract them.

Saying "mmm", or making other supportive sounds: If used from time to time in appropriate places, this shows that you are listening, and that you are actively engaged.

Leaning forward toward them: This shows that you are involved and concerned. It is as if you are symbolically reaching out to them.

Checking you have understood

"Paraphrasing" is another active listening skill, which counsellors learn. It involves repeating what you have heard, but in your own words.

It's helpful to use this skill for the important things that your friend or loved one has said – the key messages from what they are telling you.

What this does:

- It shows the other person that you have *processed* what they said – that you are *trying to understand* (because you are using your own words, not just repeating their words).
- It allows you to *check your understanding of the facts* – to ensure you have understood what they are telling you.
- It gives them the chance to correct you, if you have not quite understood what they are trying to explain.

If you use paraphrasing to reflect back the *feelings* they have expressed, not just the facts or events they have described, it is even more effective.

EXAMPLE SITUATION

This is a situation where someone is unable to leave their home, and they are communicating a) what has led up to this and b) how this makes them feel:

Your friend or neighbour explains that she was randomly attacked in the street a few weeks ago, and her purse/handbag was stolen. This has left her feeling fearful of leaving her home. She is afraid to leave her safe space. Her doctor thinks she may have developed a phobia of going out (agoraphobia), as a result of this.

You might paraphrase this in a conversation with her by saying something like:

"I can hear that you have been through something really traumatic. Being attacked in the street by a stranger has left you feeling very frightened – and particularly afraid to leave your home."

Reflecting their feelings/emotions back to them

This is a really important skill when you are supporting someone – it can make such a difference. If you only remember one of the listening skills from this chapter, I would be delighted if this is the one.

Empathy is about understanding what someone is feeling *from their frame of reference* (not what you may feel in similar circumstances).

When you are listening to your friend or family member, try to pick up on the feelings that they are expressing. They may be feeling angry or confused – or afraid, like the woman in the example I just gave. They may be feeling deep distress or profound emotional pain. They may feel overwhelmed. Conversely, they may be feeling numb or detached and disconnected – a lack of emotion. This can happen after a very painful or shocking event, for example.

If you "reflect back" that emotion to them, it can be incredibly powerful. This means you say back the emotion or feeling in your own words. Sometimes you will hear them reply with an emphatic "yes", because they feel that you really get what they are feeling. It can make such a difference to them feeling understood. It shows empathy, which is so important.

Empathy can be so helpful when they are explaining the circumstances that have led up to their crisis: recent life events that may have been distressing for them.

Using the phrase "It sounds like you are feeling..." can be helpful, e.g. "It sounds like you are feeling really frightened." This allows them to correct you, if you haven't got it quite right.

EXAMPLE SITUATION

I'm going to return to the situation I have just described, where someone is afraid to leave their home because of a recent attack in the street.

You've already reflected back the fear she is experiencing. She goes on to explain more about how it feels:

"I feel like a prisoner here. I feel so alone. I never see anyone."

If we focus carefully on the words she is saying, we might give this kind of reply:

"It sounds like you are feeling really isolated and trapped at home." **Really isolated** (picking up on the "alone" and "not seeing anyone") and **trapped at home** (picking up on the word "prisoner").

By saying these "feelings" words back using your own words, you give a strong message to your friend or loved one that you are really *hearing them, and empathizing*. And you are building a *strong connection* with them, too.

This strong connection is very important. When someone is having suicidal thoughts they may start to disconnect from the world, and from life itself, and so it is important to do all we can to build and maintain that strong connection with them.

EXAMPLE SITUATION

What Happens When You Don't See it From Their Perspective

I'm going to give an example to explain what can happen when we see things from *our* perspective, not theirs.

So this time, the same woman explains how she feels, using the same words:

"I feel like a prisoner here. I feel so alone. I never see anyone."

But when we hear this, we think about how *we* might feel in the same situation. That might be different from how they are telling us they feel. So the listener might think of all the things they would not be able to do, if they couldn't leave home. They might focus on how restrictive it would feel. This might lead them to reply, for example:

"It must be frustrating not to be able to go out when you want to."

In saying this, they are trying hard to understand. But *they are not actually reflecting back* what the woman is telling them. They are not focusing on the actual words and feelings that she is expressing.

What the woman is describing – the feeling of being a prisoner, and feeling so alone – is different from feeling frustrated.

If you don't quite get the right feeling, then they will often correct you, and explain to you what they are feeling, and this helps you to understand more.

Asking questions to understand more

There are "open" and "closed" questions. Both of these types of questions are important. They have different purposes.

Closed questions usually require a "yes" or "no" answer and/or specific information. We often use them when we need to get very precise, key information. These were the kind of questions we used to ask about suicide risk in Chapter 7, e.g. "Are you having suicidal thoughts?"

We can also use closed questions when we need to be clear and exact about something else that our friend or loved one is explaining to us.

For example, we would usually want to ask the woman who was attacked in the street: "Have you reported the crime to the police?"

However, if we are trying to encourage someone to talk or "open up" to us, then **open questions** are a good way to do this. They encourage the other person to give longer answers and disclose more information. Open questions often begin with: what, when, where, who, how, or why.

"What kind of support have you been receiving since the incident?"

"How have you been spending your days since the incident?"

This helps you to understand more about how their quality of life has been impaired since the attack.

In this situation, your visiting them can make a significant difference. It will mean a lot to them to know that you are there for them, you want to help, and they are not going to be alone. And there is good professional help available for agoraphobia.

Clinicians may recommend a treatment such as cognitive behavioural therapy (CBT). Their doctor can refer them for CBT, or advise them how to access it.

The attack in the street is a very traumatic incident, and so in these kinds of circumstances (violent and deeply shocking crimes) clinicians recommend that you do not try to draw out detailed information about the actual event, as I explained before. It can be really harrowing and distressing for someone to "re-live" the traumatic event. It's best to leave this delicate work to psychologists or psychiatric clinicians, who are trained to help someone re-live a traumatic experience safely.

KEEP PRACTISING

The techniques described in this chapter can be extremely helpful in ensuring that someone feels heard, understood and supported, and that their emotions and experiences have been validated. They can assist you in building a strong connection and empathy with the person you are concerned about. If these techniques are new to you, you'll find that you'll feel more confident and comfortable to use them the more you practise them.

9

BEYOND WORDS: BODY LANGUAGE AND OBSERVATION

In the last chapter we focused on what someone tells us with their words. But there are other ways in which people communicate with us.

BODY LANGUAGE AND VOICE TONE

Your friend or loved one may not always be able to tell you how they feel with words. But their body language and tone of voice can give powerful messages about what they are feeling. Voice tone, in particular, can express so much.

I first learned about voice tone (and what it can communicate) many years ago. That learning has always stayed with me, and it has played a vital role in my work with clients in suicidal crisis.

Over time, you can become highly attuned to slight changes in tone. When I am phoning a client to check how they are, their first two words (often simply, "Hello, Joy") may already tell me quite a lot, because of the tone of voice, and how that tone may be different from the last time we spoke. It can give an indication of their mood.

Noticing changes

Your previous knowledge of your friend, colleague or loved one allows you to pick up on any changes in their body language or the way they speak.

For example, their voice tone may have become flat, and more monotone. This can happen as someone becomes more depressed. They may make less eye contact than usual. Their posture may be different – more slumped or more closed. Or conversely, they may seem very agitated: finding it hard to stay still, and speaking faster than usual. They may make constant repetitive movements like rubbing their arms.

The changes may be smaller and more subtle, however – the better you know someone, the easier it is to pick up on slight changes. And the more you practise paying attention to people's voice tone, the more skilled you will become at this.

You probably have a much greater knowledge of your friend or family member's body language than professionals. You have probably spent much more time with them than professionals have. Professionals may only see them from time to time.

This greater knowledge was highlighted during our research into deaths by suicide. One of the families was very concerned about the suicide risk of their loved one – a young man. He had expressed suicidal thoughts the previous night, and had gone missing. When he returned home, his parents called out the family doctor. He came out to assess their son.

The doctor assessed him and concluded that he was not suicidal. His father questioned this, because he was extremely worried about his risk of suicide.

Later, the family asked the doctor if their loved one had been covering his mouth during the assessment. The doctor said that yes, he had been covering his mouth with his top. "He does that when he is not telling the truth", his family explained.

His family's knowledge of the young man's body language was so important.

We know that even people who are generally very honest may not always tell the truth about their risk of suicide. When they are not telling the truth, you may be able to tell from changes in their body language or from subtle changes to their voice tone.

Most people feel very uncomfortable about not telling the truth, and it often causes subtle changes in their voice tone.

A mismatch between words and body language

Sometimes, body language and voice tone won't match what is being said.

For example, they say "I'm fine", but their body language and voice tone seem to suggest otherwise. They may say the words in a flat, low tone. They might be hunched over, or hugging themselves tightly. Their eyes may be cast down to the floor.

There are many reasons why they may say "I'm fine", when they're not. They may not be able to face talking to anyone at the moment. They may be scared to tell people how they really feel; they may be afraid of how people will react. They may be too exhausted to talk (particularly if they are depressed – talking can be exhausting when you are deeply depressed). Or perhaps they feel they can't let anyone in at the moment. Perhaps they worry that no one will understand.

It can help to be gentle but persistent when someone tells you they are "fine". We want to be respectful of their need for space – if they are feeling exhausted or overwhelmed and are finding it hard to be around people – but we are concerned about them, because they don't seem fine at all. You could say: "I'm concerned because you seem very low."

If they are reluctant to talk further, you can simply ask: "Is it okay if I sit with you for a while?" Being able to sit with them – even if it is in silence – can be a first step in the connection process. Just by being there, you are showing your concern and care. If you feel someone is closing themselves off from you and other people, being present beside them sends an important message.

What we see: Other visual clues

It is not just someone's body language that provides us with important information. Changes in their appearance may tell us something about their mood, too. If they start to take less care of their appearance, it may be a sign that they are becoming more depressed, for example. When you are depressed it becomes much harder to care for yourself.

However, it is important to dispel the myth that someone who is "well dressed" and "well kempt" is less at risk of suicide. Many people with strong suicidal thoughts or a plan to end their life continue to dress smartly and take great care of their appearance.

When someone is masking their suicide risk

Some people who are having suicidal thoughts – or are planning to end their life – may appear to many people as if they are "okay". We know that some clients at our Suicide Crisis Centre are very reluctant to tell family or friends. They work very hard at presenting to other people as if they are okay. We do all we can to encourage them to share their thoughts with their loved ones, but sometimes they still feel unable to do so.

Presenting as though they are okay can be utterly exhausting for them. The constant effort needed to cover up their profound emotional pain and distress can make things even harder for them – it can place a huge strain on them, and can deplete their inner reserves massively.

People might think: "How could I not have known that they were having such strong suicidal thoughts? I didn't see anything that made me think that."

It is possible for some people to cover up their suicidal feelings very well. I think this is partly because many of us become skilled at covering up our feelings from early adulthood onward – often because we have to, in order to be able to function well at work, or in other situations.

There may be deeply distressing things happening in our personal lives – the terminal illness of a family member, or a family bereavement, for example. But we go to work, and in order to do our work well, we may present to the outside world as if we are completely fine. This "learning to function well when we are in emotional pain" means that when we experience a suicidal crisis, we may be able to put on a front, and seem entirely "okay" to most people.

In later chapters I will focus on what can be helpful when you are worried about someone but they are shutting you out.

HOW DO WE ADDRESS THE WIDER ISSUE OF "NO WARNING SIGNS"?

In terms of people masking their suicidal feelings, and not showing some of the "warning signs" that might alert you to their risk, we know that men are much less likely than women to talk about their emotions to each other. In recent years, mental health charities have run campaigns to urge people to "ask twice" how their friends and family members are. We so often tell our friends that we are "okay" when in reality, we may be struggling or indeed we may be in mental health crisis. So people are encouraged to ask a second time: "How are you really?"

If you're a man and you feel able to talk to your male friends about your own mental health, you are likely to encourage them to feel that they can do the same. For example: "I've had times in my life when I've felt really depressed. I think it's important to feel able to talk about it."

Perhaps we can also take opportunities to talk about suicide more generally, before our help is needed. So when we watch a documentary about suicide online or on television, or we read a relevant book, it can provide opportunities to raise the subject.

For example: "I was watching a documentary about suicide online/reading a book about suicide prevention and it made me think about the subject. It's not something people talk about much – even to close friends and family. People can feel frightened to talk about it. I was watching/reading how people who are feeling suicidal may feel they can't tell anyone – they try to protect their family and friends, or they feel they can't tell them for some other reason. I just wanted to say that if you ever felt that you wanted to end your life, I would always rather know and have the chance to help. I would always be here for you."

10

BARRIERS TO CONNECTING

I'm going to focus on things that can get in the way of you connecting with your friend or family member. As I explained in Chapter 1, it's very understandable if you feel complex emotions upon learning that someone you know is feeling suicidal. But by responding in some of the ways I describe in this chapter, you could cause your friend or family member to distance themselves from you. So I'm going to explain alternative ways of responding, which will help you to keep connected with them.

CRITICIZING OR DISMISSING THEIR FEELINGS

Some clients at our Suicide Crisis Centre have felt criticized by people close to them when they are in crisis. It has been so upsetting for them if they have spoken about their feelings, and family members or friends respond by saying that they are "being dramatic" or "over-dramatizing their feelings".

This often leads to the person disconnecting from the friend or family member. Their emotional pain or distress is not being acknowledged, and instead of being supported or comforted, they are being criticized.

Only they themselves really know how they are feeling. *It is not for us to know or judge how much feeling is "enough" or "too much"*. If they tell us that something has happened that feels acutely painful, then it is so important that we hear this, empathize and reflect this back (as described in Chapter 8).

> None of us can fully know the depth of someone else's emotional pain. The fact that someone else cannot imagine feeling such pain in a similar situation simply shows that we are all different. To feel things deeply should not be seen as something negative.

People who feel things deeply are usually extremely empathic, caring, sensitive, loving individuals – and these are all things to celebrate.

It is also really painful if a friend or loved one suggests that feeling suicidal is an *over-reaction* to a situation.

When something is outside our own experience or imagination: dismissing the impact of incidents or their account of events

One of our clients told a family member that she was being bullied at work. She described some of the incidents to them. They reacted by saying: "I can understand that kind of thing happening in the police force or the army – but surely it wouldn't be happening in your line of work."

In saying this, her family member gave the impression that she doubted her experience of being bullied. It was extremely distressing to feel not believed. When a friend or loved one discloses something like this, *it is so important that their experience is acknowledged*. When she finally spoke to a professional who immediately accepted and believed her account of events to be the truth, it was hugely powerful, she explained. It was the start of being able to process what had happened to her.

Another client described being stalked – a terrifying experience for her. Some members of her family found it hard to accept that what she described was stalking. She only described a few of the recent events to them. Taken in isolation, some of the incidents may have seemed like small acts. But when you put them together, they formed a pattern of behaviour, which amounted to stalking. Stalking is about fixation and obsession.

Sometimes, when something is outside our own experience, it can be hard, initially, to grasp its likely impact on someone else. I recall a client at our Suicide Crisis Centre describing how he had recently been through a disciplinary process at work, because he had allegedly broken one of the fundamental rules at work.

"The disciplinary process felt violent", he commented, at one point. I remember feeling momentarily surprised because he was using the word "violent" to describe how the disciplinary process felt to him. For a moment, the choice of word was unexpected, in the context. I am much more used to hearing it to describe actual acts of physical harm. *But this was about how it had felt to him.*

"It sounds like it felt brutal to you", I suggested. "Yes, that's it exactly!" he replied immediately.

As we continued to talk, it was clear that he felt psychologically damaged by the experience, and I was able to reflect that back to him. This was highlighted in his initial description of the process as "violent". He had been wrongly accused of serious misconduct, based on the witness account of a member of staff he had previously trusted. He was accused of things that went against his own moral code.

> The more we learn about a person's situation and experience, the more we are likely to be able to understand and empathize.

FEELING THAT PERSON HAS CHANGED BEYOND RECOGNITION – THAT YOU DON'T KNOW THEM ANYMORE

It can be a shock for friends and family to see someone they know in suicidal crisis, especially if they have never experienced this before. "Suddenly, it's like they are a different person – this is not the person I know", one family member commented. Sometimes, family members distance themselves from the person in crisis, because they don't seem like the same person anymore.

When someone is in suicidal crisis or mentally unwell (for example, depressed) they may seem very different from usual. They may not be able to function in the way they used to, because *their illness has taken over for a period of time.*

They may also act very differently during this period. So, in many ways, they are "not themselves" at this time. But they are still *fundamentally that same person you know.* They have not lost the wonderful unique qualities that make them who they are. Maybe you can't see that at the moment – it's as if their depression or mental illness has taken over for a period of time – but they are still there.

When someone is in suicidal crisis, they may feel that they are no longer the person that they were. This can feel very distressing. If they are depressed, for example, they may find it very hard to see that this could be temporary. They may assume that this change in them is permanent and that "the old me has gone forever". It is important that we give them the message that they are still themselves: "You are still you – you are still the mum/dad/sister/brother that we love so much."

I remember when one of our clients called us, very distressed. He had smashed all the cups in his flat. He had never done anything like this before – he had never damaged property. He saw this as a sign that he was not the person he used to be. But he was deeply depressed, and his depression was influencing his behaviour. This was of course really concerning in terms of increased suicide risk, because smashing crockery showed a loss of control over his actions. I will talk about anger again in Chapter 14.

It is of course really painful for you to see such a significant change in your family member or friend. Please do seek support for yourself. Although we provide crisis services for people who are at risk of suicide, it is so important that we are there for the family members and friends of our clients in crisis, too. You can seek support from local services or national helplines, and there is more information about accessing support for yourself in Chapter 17.

TALKING IN TERMS OF STRENGTH AND WEAKNESS

It can be a particularly difficult adjustment when the person in crisis is someone who family or friends have relied on a lot in the past – perhaps the person who has always been there for everyone else.

It can lead family members or friends to express their dismay. They may say things like: "But you're a strong person!" or "You're the strong one!"

Feeling suicidal is not a sign that someone has become "weak" or "weaker", though. It is not about strength and weakness. They are in crisis at the moment, and need to be supported and cared for until they recover. A suicidal crisis can happen to anyone, including the bravest of us.

It is interesting to see how often the message, "Stay strong!" is sent to people who are in crisis. We often see it posted on social media when someone says they are struggling. I have always found this difficult to understand because it seems to send a message that they should rely on themselves and depend on their own resources. It seems to promote self-reliance.

I would much rather see friends writing comments like: "I am here for you", and "Please keep talking to us" – messages that emphasize that they want to support and help.

> Rather than "staying strong", we really want people to *feel able to be vulnerable* and share their feelings, not suppress them and carry on.

COMPARING THEIR CIRCUMSTANCES TO SOMEONE ELSE'S SITUATION

Sometimes friends and family may struggle to understand why someone is feeling suicidal and may make comments such as: "But you have a great life!" or "There are so many other people worse off than you" or even, "Think about all the people in the world who are suffering far more than you."

I remember a family member of one of our clients said to him: "You should count yourself lucky that you have reached your sixties and never had a suicidal crisis before. I felt suicidal when I was in my thirties. Some people feel suicidal in their teens."

The younger family member was in fact really supportive and she helped her older family member enormously through his suicidal crisis. Indeed, the fact that she had experienced suicidal crisis herself was partly why he felt able to open up to her. But he found this comparison made him feel guilty about his depression and suicidal feelings – and ashamed about how low he was feeling: "I should not be feeling this. There are other people worse off than me."

> It is important that we give a message that *their feelings are valid* and their pain and suffering is legitimate.

JUDGING BASED ON RELIGIOUS BELIEFS

I have huge respect for the different religious faiths. Many people find their own faith helps them enormously during a time of crisis. And they often receive exceptional support from their place of worship or members of the congregation.

However, sometimes friends or family members who have strong religious beliefs have been known to chastise the person who is in suicidal crisis. They have made comments that feeling suicidal is sinful. This can be really distressing for the person in crisis. It is not for me to question anyone's religious beliefs about what constitutes a sin. But there is a risk that the person could feel cast out by their religion. It could also increase negative feelings that they may already have about themselves. And for someone who was not previously religious, but may have turned to God at this time, it might make them feel that they have no right to do so.

It's important to stress that many people who have a deep religious conviction would take a different approach. Their view is that their loving God embraces the person who is struggling with a suicidal crisis, recognizing their suffering and pain. When someone is very vulnerable and in crisis, love (which is at the heart of religions) and unconditional support is likely to be so much more helpful and effective.

WHEN SOMETHING GOES AGAINST OUR MORAL CODE

It can be very hard to know how to respond when we hear that a friend or family member has done something we could not condone, or something that goes against our beliefs or moral code.

For example, they may tell you that they have committed a crime and are under investigation by the police. Or you may find that they have been having an affair. This may now be impacting on their risk of suicide. They may have overwhelming feelings of guilt and regret. They may also be dealing with the consequences – a possible criminal record or, in the case of an affair, the loss of the relationship.

Understandably, you may have very strong feelings about this. It's understandable that you would feel deeply upset for the people who have been directly affected: the victims of the crime, or in the case of an affair, the partner of the family member or friend. You might feel a huge loyalty to the partner in the relationship.

It can help to try to separate the person from what they have done.

It doesn't mean you approve of what they have done or that you overlook it. It doesn't mean you think it's okay. But you still care deeply about them as a person and you are still really concerned about them. You can still support them.

It can help to find out more about the circumstances. There are often complex reasons why something has happened. Sometimes, a person who is becoming mentally unwell (or descending into crisis) may act very differently from usual. Again, this is not an attempt to excuse what has happened, but rather to understand more about what may have led to it.

> Supporting someone through this can be so hard for you – you may be experiencing very complex emotions. It may feel really painful for you. This is one of the many situations where it is so important that *you also have access to support,* to help you with the painful and conflicting feelings you may have.

TELLING SOMEONE TO "GET OVER IT"

Recently, I was asking a client at our Suicide Crisis Centre whether he was receiving any support from family or friends. He said that one of his parents had taken quite some time to recognize the impact of depression on him. At first, his father's view was that he should be able to "snap out of it". Our client said: "I don't think he realized that it was hard enough to get out of bed in the morning. I couldn't magically make myself better."

As time has gone by, his father has read and learned more about depression and our client finds his approach has changed; it is much more supportive and helpful now.

Other phrases like this include: "Pull yourself together", and "You need to sort yourself out."

Learning more about the complexity of suicidal crisis can help people to understand why it is just not possible for someone to be able to wish themselves better.

11

WHAT TO FOCUS ON

This chapter looks at helpful things you can say to someone during a period of suicidal crisis.

CELEBRATING THEIR POSITIVE QUALITIES

I've explained how *someone in suicidal crisis may have lost sight of their own worth*, particularly if they are deeply depressed. Depression can make a person feel that they have nothing to offer the world. Depression can attack someone's sense of self-worth, shattering their self-esteem. It's so important that we remind them of everything that makes them so precious and unique – all their wonderful qualities. There is no one else like them.

From the early days of providing services at our Suicide Crisis Centre, I was struck by the wonderful qualities we saw in our clients. These individual qualities shone out. They were some of the most caring, giving individuals you could wish to meet. But often, they did not know this. These qualities were so obvious to us, but they could not see them.

When we tell someone about the qualities we see in them, they sometimes reject what we say. It can be hard for them to believe it. They sometimes think we are just being kind. So it can be helpful to give them some evidence to back up what we are saying.

We point out things they have said to us (or things they have done), which provide evidence of this positive quality.

For example, one of our clients was convinced that he was only a "negative presence". "There's a darkness inside me", he used to say. "It's better that I keep away from people – that I don't see anyone." He had severe PTSD after losing members of his family in a violent accident. He had experienced both severe trauma and heartbreaking loss. Since the accident, he had struggled with overwhelming feelings of anger at times, and rages which he found hard to control. One day, his daughter had told him: "You scare me." That was a defining moment for him. He felt that he should remove himself from other people. He isolated himself and stopped seeing friends or family.

It was clear that he had never had psychological therapy to help him to process the severe trauma and loss of family members, and this was going to be important to help address the rage he felt inside. But in the meantime, we could gently challenge his perception of himself as a "negative force".

We saw so much evidence of his good qualities. I remember one day how he messaged me because he had just seen a news report about people who were suffering. He felt such a profound empathy for other people who were experiencing emotional or physical pain. And on another day, I was talking on the phone to him, and I suddenly heard another voice. He explained: "I'll have to go." He explained that an elderly woman from across the road couldn't get into her house. The door was stuck and she had come to ask him for help.

I pointed out to him later that his neighbour clearly trusted him – and this was significant. Out of all her neighbours on the estate, she had come to *him* at a time when she was very vulnerable. She did not see him as frightening or a threat – indeed, the opposite. She saw him as trustworthy and a source of safety. And of course, his immediate wish to help someone in need was clear evidence of his caring nature.

Highlighting an individual's personal qualities is about *their innate worth, aside from anything they contribute to the world* (through their paid work or voluntary work, for example). It is important to emphasize that they have innate worth, which is not linked to what they achieve or accomplish in life.

HIGHLIGHTING HOW THEY MAKE A DIFFERENCE

Although not as important as our innate worth, it can also help to remind someone of what they contribute to the world: how they help their friends, how they care about the people around them, how they enhance life for other people, for example.

This is not so much about achievements or accomplishments, but about *how their existence makes a difference to the world.*

They may also provide meaningful contributions through creative pursuits: through their art or writing and how other people can appreciate these and derive pleasure from them, or can be challenged by or learn from them.

They may contribute through their work (paid or voluntary). It is not only through the obvious helping professions that people can make such a difference. In any job which involves contact with other people, we have an impact. One of our clients works in stock control. It became clear that other members of staff always seemed to confide in her, when they were going through difficult times. Even when she was going through her own crisis, she still worried about her colleagues at work, who she knew were also going through their own difficulties.

THE POWERFUL HUMAN INSTINCT TO HELP OTHER PEOPLE

I remember one of the police officers who we supported, and how intense her suicidal thoughts were, at times. One evening, she was having strong thoughts of ending her life. However, she spoke about a boy who she had met recently in the course of her work. He had been badly bullied. She had made a commitment to go back and talk to him the following day. It was of course partly a strong sense of duty that ensured she kept that commitment. But it was also that he mattered very much. It mattered that she kept that commitment. She knew that her contribution to his wellbeing and recovery could make a difference to him.

That instinct to help other people in need often remains strong even when someone is having powerful thoughts of suicide. I have seen it so many times. I have seen it happen in an Emergency Department in a hospital. A woman was there because she was at immediate risk of suicide. She heard someone nearby who was clearly in mental anguish. Her immediate thought was that she wanted to comfort them, despite her own profound distress.

It is such a beautiful aspect of human nature. I often say that we see the very best of human nature at our Suicide Crisis Centre.

EXPLORING WHAT MAKES LIFE MEANINGFUL FOR THEM

For many of us, it is our family or friends who make life meaningful for us. But many people don't have such meaningful connections in their life. Not everyone comes from a supportive family. Those of us who were fortunate enough to have a loving family may now be separated from them through death, divorce or loss of custody. This may be part of what is contributing to someone's suicidal crisis. So it can be important to look wider than close personal relationships when trying to help someone to see meaning in their life.

As we have seen in so many of our clients, helping other people is one of the things that makes life meaningful. It is what clients most often say to us when they are starting to recover from their suicidal crisis: "I just want to help as many people as I can in the future." For many people, this is a very powerful reason to live. For some of us, it is one of the fundamental reasons why we think we are here on Earth.

As we get to know our clients at the Suicide Crisis Centre, it becomes clear that many of them also want to change things for the better. They want to make the world a better place in some way for other people. It is why they eventually become involved in charities that focus on battling against injustices, or those that alleviate suffering in some way.

It's important to stress that they may not feel that they can do any of these things at the moment – because they are in crisis. It is more about *re-connecting them with the concept of the things that matter to them.*

And it is of course very individual. It's about finding out what they care about – what they are passionate about when they are not in crisis.

For one of our clients, it was martial arts. When he came to us first, he was adamant that there was nothing to live for. He told us that he had no personal connections. His relationship had just ended. He not only saw no hope for himself, he said, but he also saw no hope for the world in general. So I asked him: "What has made your life meaningful in the past?"

Of course, his relationship with his ex-partner had made life extremely meaningful, but it was about looking beyond that to see what else mattered to him.

He immediately mentioned this particular martial art. I had never heard of it, and wanted to know more. He explained how it was really inclusive: "Anyone can do it – literally anyone", he said. He felt that the mental health benefits were really significant. He spoke about "stress relief", "the meditative aspect", and how "calming" he found it. He felt that so many people could benefit from it. He clearly had a desire for other people to have the opportunity to do it. He felt it could help them in the same way that it had helped him in the past.

I wanted other people to know about it too, and we explored how he could write about his experience for our next newsletter, which reaches hundreds of people. He started to think about other ways he could raise awareness of the martial art – particularly for people with mental health issues.

Up until then, the young man had spoken very little to me. He had remained quite disconnected. This martial art gave me a way to connect with him: I was genuinely interested to learn more about the benefits.

> We can often find ways of connecting with someone through the things in life which matter most to them: their passion in life or what makes life meaningful for them.

For another of our clients, it was her dog. She had such a strong bond with him. I recall one night when she was designated a high-risk missing person by the police. It was my first contact with her. One of her family members had phoned us to explain that she was missing and at risk of suicide. They asked us to try to contact her. The family member later sent us a message: "Talk to her about her dog." It was excellent advice. They knew how much he mattered to her. It was a powerful way to connect with her. It meant that she engaged with me, and we were able to communicate with each other until the police were able to reach her.

CONNECTING TO THE PART OF THEM THAT WANTS TO SURVIVE

Some counsellors, when working with someone in suicidal crisis, talk about "working with the part of them that wants to survive". Friends and family members may want to consider using this phrase, too.

This can be helpful to some people in crisis, because it gives full recognition of the fact that the bigger part of them may want to end their life. It is often reassuring to them that this bigger part is fully acknowledged.

This approach also highlights (to the person in crisis) that there is still a small part of them that is trying to survive. They may not have actually fully realized or acknowledged this until now. It's the part of them that is allowing you to support them (and involve professional help).

Their grip on life may be very tenuous, but we are still holding on tightly to that tiny part of them that wants to survive.

REMINDING THEM IT WILL NOT ALWAYS BE THIS WAY

It can help to reassure your friend or family member that it will not always be this way. Life will not always be as it is now. It always changes. This may of course be incredibly hard for them to absorb or accept.

This is not the same as saying that "suicide is a permanent solution to a temporary problem". This is a popular phrase on suicide prevention websites. It is extremely well-meaning. But it assumes that the factors that have led to a suicidal crisis are temporary. It may even suggest that they are short-lived. Some people feel that this minimizes what they are experiencing.

Some of the factors which can lead to a suicidal crisis are longer term – serious physical health problems, for example, and profound grief. If you have lost someone close to you, it can feel acutely painful to feel it is being dismissed as a "temporary problem".

Life can improve and be very different in the future, even after immense suffering – and even in the midst of suffering. There may be ways to alleviate physical suffering – sometimes we can help our friend or loved one to access different treatments. And someone's quality of life can improve, for example through new people they meet in the future, or new things they become involved with. Their physical condition may not have changed, but their life has changed. That can help to make their physical health symptoms more bearable.

Someone who is completely alone now may form meaningful connections in the future.

Life always has the power to surprise us, and to bring things or people into our life that we did not expect.

This is why the phrase "life will not always be as it is now" can be helpful, because it focuses more on the possibility of positive life changes in the future, but does not suggest that the intense and prolonged pain of grief is "temporary" or short-term.

Although they may not feel able to believe that their acute suffering could be alleviated, or that their circumstances could change, the fact that *you* believe it can make a difference to some people.

"HOLDING THE HOPE" FOR THEM

It can be profoundly moving when someone offers to "hold the hope for you", or "carry the hope for you". Counsellors sometimes use this phrase. It can mean different things to different people.

It is a phrase you can use when your friend or loved one has told you that they have no hope for the future: "I can hear that you feel you have no hope, so I am going to carry the hope for you, as we walk forward on this journey together."

It can be a way of saying that you will be connected with them throughout their crisis. It is as if you are walking alongside them on their journey, carrying the hope that they cannot carry for themselves at the moment. It links you throughout the time that you are supporting them.

It also symbolizes that hope is not lost (which is what the person in crisis may think). It still exists.

It is different from saying, "There is hope" – which is offering the direct opposite of what they are thinking. This can be hard for them to absorb or accept, at that point.

> An offer to hold the hope for them introduces the concept of hope more gently. And it shows your personal commitment to them.

12

KINDNESS, COMPASSION AND CARE

Caring and kindness have such a powerful effect when someone is in suicidal crisis. I cannot emphasize this enough. It is why your involvement can make such a difference.

KINDNESS AND CARE

When someone is in suicidal crisis, they may disconnect from the people around them. They may do this consciously or unconsciously. It may be part of the preparation for ending their life – trying to detach from the people they love. They may place a barrier around themselves, to keep people out. In that detached place, they can be very much at risk.

Kindness has the power to break through this barrier. It is so hard not to respond to a kind, caring approach. It is very hard to shut out kindness. It is utterly disarming.

There is no doubt that kindness can be life-saving. We should never underestimate its power. It is one of the most important things you can offer, when you are trying to help someone to survive a suicidal crisis. Your caring will help more than you will ever know.

KEEPING CONNECTED IN AS MANY WAYS AS POSSIBLE

Helping someone to stay connected is so important. If they seem to be rejecting offers to meet or to talk on the phone, then texting, emailing, and sending letters or cards are other ways to keep connected. This is a way for friends and family to show very clearly that they care about them, and are concerned.

THE POWER OF A SIMPLE TEXT

I know from personal experience how powerful text messages can be from someone you know, who clearly cares about you. In a depressive episode, I stopped communicating with people, including friends. One of my friends decided to text me three times a day: in the morning, the middle of the day, and in the evening.

If someone had asked me at the time whether my friend texting me was making a difference, I would have replied that I didn't think so. I was so profoundly depressed and disconnected, and life had lost all its meaning. I didn't have any feeling that it made things any better. However, when I was recovering from my depression, I realized that it had indeed had an impact, even though I could not recognize it at the time. It meant that I was never alone. He was walking alongside me the whole time. Someone who cared about me very much was always present.

So, *even if you are getting very little response from the person you are messaging, there are very good reasons to continue to do it.* It is very likely that it will have an impact – even if the person receiving it doesn't realize it.

One of our clients was very reluctant to see family members, even though they really wanted to help. It was partly because his depression left him so exhausted, and partly because he didn't want his family to see him depressed. So they came up with a plan to help. The different family members focused on providing food. They knew he had always liked his food, when he was well.

His sister would cook a Sunday lunch and take a portion round to him. She didn't stay if he didn't feel up to it, but her delivery of food was in itself an expression of love and care.

Another day, a different family member would cook a curry and take a couple of portions for him, one to eat and one for the freezer. On Fridays and Saturdays, his nephew would order one of his favourite takeaways.

Although he found it hard to spend time with family, this was a way his loved ones could express their care for him. Providing food has so many connections with nurturing and caring. And of course they were doing something really important, in terms of his mental wellbeing. When someone is depressed, they may find it hard to prepare meals or to eat much. And a lack of food really impacts on mood. Getting good nourishment is so important during a period of crisis.

HELPING WITH THE FACTORS THAT HAVE LED TO THEIR CRISIS

When we first started seeing clients at our Suicide Crisis Centre, we found that we were doing more than supporting them emotionally. We found ourselves instinctively trying to help them with aspects of their life that were causing them pain. These were often aspects of their life that were impacting on their suicide risk.

When one of our clients was going through a disciplinary process at work, for example, we were able to help in some practical ways. He was convinced that he was going to lose his job, and believed that he would not get another one, with this disciplinary matter on his record. It was clear that he had been a valued employee with an exemplary record up until a few months previously. At that point, his mental health had deteriorated as a result of increased stresses at work. He had been working long night shifts and the work had been very emotionally demanding. He became sleep-deprived. He was mentally and physically exhausted, probably to the point of burnout. He had also become very depressed. Sadly, burnout often tips into depression. When he broke the rules, there were many mitigating circumstances. There were other factors contributing to his suicidal crisis, but this was a factor which was causing his risk of suicide to escalate.

We helped him with his statement for the disciplinary process, because he was finding it so hard to think clearly and write it himself. Additionally, we accompanied him to the disciplinary hearing, to support him. Fortunately, managers recognized the mitigating factors, and he kept his job. However, we had also spent time helping him to look at other ways forward, in case he lost his job. And the fact that he was supported throughout the disciplinary process made a difference, he said. He knew that we really cared – our genuine wish to help showed him that.

Another of our clients (Amelia) had lost custody of her younger children to her ex-husband. This was heartbreaking for her. In the family court, her ex-husband argued that her mental health was a factor that meant she should not care for them. She had been deeply depressed for a period of time. But many, many devoted parents experience depression.

It was important that we helped and supported Amelia to have more access to her children. The family court judge required her to take a parenting course before she could see her children more frequently. But she needed literacy support to do it. She hadn't wanted to tell the judge this. We were very fortunate that one of our team was a qualified English teacher, who had taught adult literacy classes in the past. Our client trusted her, and she was able to support her to complete the course.

Amelia had lost confidence in her ability to be a parent, because of the family court judgment. Her parenting abilities had been called into question during the court process. Her self-worth was severely affected. So we knew that we needed to help her to know that she was a good parent.

While we were supporting Amelia, we got to know her older children, who were in their late teens. All of them were compassionate, responsible young people, who were clearly respected by their teachers and employers. We pointed out to Amelia that they provided powerful evidence that she had excellent parenting abilities. She was a loving, devoted mother who had instilled in her children qualities that meant they were a credit to her. We also helped Amelia to provide evidence to the court of her parenting ability. As part of that, we wrote to the judge. One of the important parts of that letter to the court was to leave the judge in no doubt that Amelia's older children were powerful evidence of her excellent parenting skills.

WHAT YOU CAN DO TO HELP

In sharing this, I would not want you to feel under pressure to do things to try to alleviate your friend or family member's situation. Supporting someone in suicidal crisis is already demanding so much from you. However, there may be small things that you feel able to do, which can help. Doing research can be extremely helpful and much of this can be done online. You can find helpful websites or information relating to some of the issues that are causing them distress. And accompanying your friend or loved one to important appointments or meetings really makes a difference.

13

HELPING SOMEONE TO SURVIVE

When you are helping someone to survive a suicidal crisis, it's important that you know that you don't have to be the one to "heal them". It's the role of professionals to help with the longer-term underlying reasons for their crisis.

But one of the really important things you can do is to *help them to stay alive until they reach a point where they themselves are more able to survive.* When someone is in suicidal crisis, it is often the case that their inner resources have been profoundly depleted – perhaps because they have had to endure immensely challenging experiences or adverse life events over a prolonged period of time – and they are now struggling to survive. They need time and support while they gradually start to recover their inner resources. You can help and support them to get through the critical phase, when they are at their most vulnerable and depleted.

In this chapter we will look at some of the most effective ways you can do that.

DELAYING

You can ask someone to *delay* ending their life. Some people in crisis are willing to do this. They may be willing to accept professional help or crisis support for a period of time.

If you ask them to *commit to living*, that can feel too much for them. But asking them to wait does feel possible for some people. It may be that they feel able to commit to delaying, because it feels more short-term and manageable. In contrast, the prospect of their whole life stretching before them can feel unmanageable at the present time. So they may find it hard to agree to live, even though that is the outcome we are seeking. Delaying gives time for things to change and for their suicidal feelings to subside.

If someone is having strong thoughts of ending their life, waiting 24 hours can be life-saving. Waiting 24 hours can feel possible and manageable for many people.

When you ask them to wait, they may feel, "Yes, I could wait until tomorrow – a delay of 24 hours makes no difference."

The reality is that this 24-hour delay can be enough to *reduce their risk just enough to ensure that they survive*. Their suicidal feelings may not be quite so intense the next day. Many people attempt suicide while they are experiencing overwhelming emotions and intense inner turmoil. Their emotional turmoil has reached a peak. These very high levels of distress cloud their thinking. There may have been a final trigger, which has been really destabilizing.

Asking them to wait is *not an alternative to getting emergency crisis help* for them. It's important to immediately call for professional help, too. But you have planted the idea of waiting in their mind. This delay of 24 hours has been life-saving for many people.

> Many suicide attempts are impulsive, rather than planned. Delaying allows time for these intense feelings to subside just a little.

It is not that their suicide risk disappears after 24 hours, of course. They will still need a high level of support. But it can be just enough to reduce the risk from a critical level.

In reality, we want the person to delay for much longer – indefinitely – but we may need to move toward this gradually. We may need to create manageable steps.

As our research into deaths by suicide revealed, a significant number of people ended their life in the hours – or minutes – following a major argument. Intense emotions (including anger) can be destabilizing enough to trigger a suicide attempt.

There are other ways in which you can delay. Sometimes, family members take their loved one to an Emergency Department when they are at immediate risk of suicide. Even if the outcome is that they return home a few hours later, *this delay may have been enough to prevent a suicide attempt on this occasion.* Those hours sitting in the Emergency Department may have allowed their immediate risk to subside.

HELPING THEM TO JUST FOCUS ON TODAY

For someone in suicidal crisis, the future may seem utterly overwhelming. The prospect of continuing to live is so hard.

Focusing on the current day can help as a strategy for the medium term, over the coming weeks, until they are out of crisis. It means that the person in crisis doesn't need to think about the future. "Today" can feel more manageable than the long-term.

Some people think of it as "stepping out of time". They find that it releases them from all the demands, pressures and expectations that may have become so overwhelming.

They can do whatever they want – anything that feels helpful and manageable to them.

We can help to make today as bearable as possible for the person, too. Encouraging self-care is part of that, and doing things that are known to have positive benefits for mental health, such as spending time in nature.

When I say "self-care", I mean *anything that soothes and comforts them.*

It is absolutely okay to rest as much as possible, if that feels helpful to them. One of our clients (who is deeply depressed) often finds it really hard to find the motivation to do much at all. This is very understandable. At these times, he listens to gospel music: "I bet it surprises you that a big, tough man like me listens to gospel music", he told me. For him it is not the religious aspect that helps him. It is because it is so uplifting, he says, and so comforting. What comforts us during our darkest times can be so individual.

SPENDING TIME IN NATURE

Now that they are focused on making the present day as bearable as possible, encouraging them to spend some of the day in nature can be very helpful.

Research has shown that nature has a positive impact on mental health. But less has been written about how it can help someone to survive a suicidal crisis.

The person in crisis may have isolated themselves from other people. Perhaps you are the only person they are willing to see. *Being connected to the natural world is another way of keeping connected to the living world – and therefore to life itself.* It's about *feeling part of the natural world.* They may struggle to feel part of the "human world" at the moment.

> Nature accepts and embraces us unconditionally. We always have our place in nature, even if we feel that we have lost our place in the human world at this time.

Many of us feel a connection to the creatures we encounter as we walk in nature, whether it's the birds we can hear singing, the farm animals in the fields we pass, or squirrels scurrying quickly up a tree and rabbits rushing for cover. Even watching nature programmes on television can have a positive impact.

BECOMING ABSORBED IN SOMETHING

This involves focusing on something that takes their mind to a different place for a while. This can take their mind away from their suffering or from their suicidal thoughts. As I said at the beginning of the chapter, part of what you are doing is to help them to stay alive long enough to get to a point, eventually, where they want to survive, or are more able to survive. You are trying to make today as bearable as possible – and each day that follows – for as long as it takes for them to start to feel a little less vulnerable and at risk.

What absorbs them will be very individual. For some people it could be spending time in the garden, tending to plants or growing things. Gently pulling up weeds or trimming branches are activities that can help to calm the mind. They don't even need a garden. Planting seeds in containers indoors can be really therapeutic. It's about nurturing and looking after something living. The shoots may start to burst above the soil within days of planting.

For other people it will be writing or drawing (or therapeutic colouring in). Being creative has many positive benefits for mental health. Creative arts can provide a way to express our feelings and emotions.

But even restful activities can help. Watching television for a period of time can allow the mind to rest. It can also take us somewhere else for a while, as we become absorbed in a documentary or drama. There are many positive benefits to watching television.

When someone is deep in crisis, or at imminent risk, they may reach a point where these strategies stop helping. During a period of crisis, someone's risk of suicide can fluctuate. So these strategies can really help at times – but it's important to understand that they may not always be appropriate when someone's risk escalates.

When an individual is highly distressed and having strong thoughts of ending their life, they may react angrily to a suggestion of going for a walk: "As if that could help!" At this point, your care and concern, and your ability to connect and empathize, will be much more effective, along with involving professionals who can provide crisis care.

Interestingly, though, one of our clients always walks to a specific place as a strategy when she is having strong thoughts of suicide. She walks from her home in an urban area, until she reaches this long country road. It is quite a steep road, which extends for a few miles. Walking helps her to release the powerful emotions that have built up to intolerable levels, she says. It also removes her from the items of risk in her home. Of course, what helps *her* could be very risky for someone else. Her experience shows, again, that what helps someone at the point of suicide can be so individual.

157

When she is on this walk, I am keeping in contact with her the whole time. If she is not speaking to me on the phone then I am texting her, so that she knows that I am with her. It is very important that she is not alone on that journey. We have built a strong connection with her already, and that connection still endures even when we are not physically with her. She has often told me afterwards that she knew we were with her the whole time, and she knew we cared about her, and this made a difference.

EXERCISE AND ACTIVITY

We know that exercise can have a positive benefit on our mental health. It has helped many people during a period of crisis. It is one of a number of very good strategies that can help. However, some people may find their usual exercise regime exhausts them, and it can help to adapt it in some way.

EXERCISE THAT ENERGIZES, NOT EXHAUSTS

One of our clients, Lily, used to swim several times a week. She tried to do the same during a period of crisis. But she found that she would sit in her car afterwards and break down in tears. By the time she arrived home, she felt utterly exhausted. This made everything seem far more overwhelming. She found that going for walks was more manageable. She was still able to exercise, but not so much that it exhausted her. Going for walks can be so beneficial.

The same can apply to other activities. Another client, Ben, first came to our Suicide Crisis Centre on a weekend. He told us that he had spent the past week throwing himself into social activities as a way of trying to occupy himself and divert his thoughts. But by the end of the week, he was exhausted, overwhelmed and struggling much more.

Activity can be so helpful – but physical or mental exhaustion can make some people more vulnerable, and can increase their risk. Being tired after exercise or activity is different from being utterly exhausted from it. Depression tends to deplete our energy reserves much quicker than usual, which is something to be mindful of.

Offering to go for a walk with a friend or family member can be helpful for other reasons, too. *It can be easier for some people to talk when they are not looking at the other person.* This is particularly true when they are talking about painful or difficult subjects.

In particular, a number of our male clients have asked to meet and go for a walk, rather than see us at our Suicide Crisis Centre. Sometimes it is just because they feel more comfortable talking without having to make eye contact. And it is a more relaxed way to be with someone. But sometimes, what they want to tell us feels embarrassing or uncomfortable to them, and the lack of eye contact makes it easier.

One of our male clients asked to meet and go for a walk for his first appointment with me. We knew that he was under investigation by the police, because we had spoken to him on the phone first. As I walked with him, he spoke very honestly about the details of the crime. He had been very concerned that I would judge him. He hadn't wanted to see my reaction while he told me what he had done. By the end of the walk, he realized that I was not going to judge him, and that I absolutely wanted to support him through this.

Walking also *creates less pressure to talk.* It allows for periods of silence, too. And if your friend or loved one does not feel up to talking, *it is a way of being there for them and being supportive, without the need to talk.*

14

SUPPORTING SOMEONE WHO IS HIGHLY DISTRESSED

People in suicidal crisis can present in many different ways. Some people will be highly distressed, and will express powerful and intense emotions, which may be hard for them to control.

RESPONDING TO ANGER

Intense anger can greatly increase someone's immediate risk of suicide. It's the *loss of control* that creates much of the risk.

Someone who never usually swears may swear profusely. Every other word may be a swear word. It's a sign that they are less in control of what they are saying – and the risk is that they are also less in control of their actions, and what they do next. If they cannot release that anger safely, they may turn it inwards and direct it toward themselves. They may harm themselves or try to take their own life, if they are already in a period of suicidal crisis.

Anger is often about something else. It's often about deep emotional pain, fear or a strong sense of injustice.

It's really important for an individual to be able to *ventilate their anger* so that they can return to a calmer state. It can help them if you *allow them to express their anger* and let them tell you why they are feeling that way.

It can help if they feel you understand why they are so angry. I have experienced clients at our Suicide Crisis Centre who are incandescent with rage. In every case, I have understood the reasons for their rage. Anger is often a justifiable response to events – or at least an understandable one.

Your supportive approach to their anger can really make a difference. A *gentle approach* can really help, too. Gentleness can help to bring down their levels of anger.

It is almost always safer for them to release the anger than to internalize it. But that anger should not be harmful to you in any way, and it should not frighten you. It is important to involve professionals if this happens. Family members have contacted us when the anger becomes about something else, and is abusive or harmful.

TRAUMA AND DISTRESS

Traumatic memories or flashbacks are intensely distressing and frightening. It can feel like the person is re-living the traumatic event. They may find it hard to distinguish between past and present when they are having flashbacks.

It can help to try to *re-orientate them back to the present,* and reassure them that they are safe now: "You are safe now (and use their name here)." "You are safe now, Anna."

Again, gentleness is so helpful when you are supporting someone who is re-living traumatic events. At a time when they may feel threatened, terrified and unsafe, your gentleness can represent the opposite of what they fear: gentleness is non-threatening, reassuring and comforting.

DISSOCIATION

Some people who have been through traumatic or very stressful events experience dissociation. Dissociation is about various forms of detachment or disconnection. They may experience some (or all) of the following:

- **Feeling disconnected from themselves:** They feel detached from themselves in some way. They may feel that they are watching themselves from the outside – as if they are on the outside, looking in. They may feel like they are standing back and observing their emotions rather than actually feeling them.
- **Feeling disconnected from the world around them:** The world around them may feel unreal. They may feel like it has a dream-like quality, or is altered in some way.
- **Having gaps in their memory (dissociative amnesia):** They may find themselves in a strange place, with no idea how they got there or why they are there. Or they

may appear to be "absent" sometimes: despite every effort to attract their attention, they may not be aware of you or of their surroundings.

Dissociation is a way that the mind protects you from emotions or memories that feel too painful. It's like your mind cuts off from the feelings or memories. But the dissociative symptoms can be frightening and confusing.

GROUNDING TECHNIQUES

Grounding techniques can help some people when they are experiencing dissociation. They can also help when someone is having flashbacks or traumatic memories, or if they are very distressed.

Grounding techniques are *ways of making someone feel very connected to their present surroundings*. Some people find that focusing on the details of things they can see around them helps. They focus on the different things they can see in the room.

Some people find it helps to *feel* their immediate surroundings and feel connected in that way – so they focus on feeling their feet against the ground. This can help them feel they are "on solid ground" – firm, stable and safe. Other people find feeling a soft blanket helps.

Other people may find a particular smell helpful – this is likely to be something very individual to them. So for example, a loved one may have given them a lavender spray and they associate it with safety and comfort. Some people were very aware of a particular smell or smells during the traumatic event that they experienced – and so a very different, reassuring smell can be helpful.

Many people use a combination of all of these techniques.

SAFE PLACE IMAGERY

Some clinicians suggest safe place imagery (or calm place imagery) to people, when they are feeling frightened or distressed.

It involves thinking of a place you associate with feeling safe, secure and peaceful. This may be somewhere you have visited in the past... or it may be an imaginary place that you create in your own mind. Many people choose a beautiful outdoor location. The idea is that you can retreat there in your mind, whenever you need to. While you are there, you focus on the different things you can see around you – all the details. Some people involve other senses as well: they focus on smell and sounds.

HUMAN TOUCH

Some people find human touch comforting and soothing when they are highly distressed. Holding someone's hand, or placing your hand gently on their arm, can be enormously supportive. But when someone is having a flashback, human touch may feel very frightening. If they feel that they are back in the trauma, they may see human touch as a threat. During a flashback, they may feel safer if you give them physical space and talk to them instead.

GENTLENESS

I have mentioned gentleness several times in this chapter. It is rarely a quality that we celebrate, but it can be so powerful when you are supporting someone in suicidal crisis.

> Gentleness is helpful in so many crisis situations: in volatile and unpredictable situations when someone is full of rage, but equally in situations where someone is silent, withdrawn and very frightened.

Gentleness can be invaluable when you are trying to connect with someone in the early stages of supporting them – a gentle tone of voice and manner. This can be particularly helpful if they have experienced the opposite from other people in the recent past – if they have experienced violence, for example. It can also make a *life-saving difference* when someone is at imminent risk of suicide, and highly distressed.

There have been a couple of occasions, in the course of my work, when I have gone to visit someone in their home and they have had a weapon in their hand that they are intending to use against themselves.

In this fragile and unpredictable situation, a gentle approach and manner can indeed make a life-saving difference. It was important that I did nothing to startle or alarm the person. I moved slowly. I spoke calmly and softly. I explained what I was doing at every stage (especially if that involved any movement) so that nothing surprised them.

It was vital that I involved emergency services. I needed to explain this to the person holding the weapon. The trust and connection that we had built with them (from our previous contact with them) played an important role at this point. They trusted me enough to believe that I had their best interests at heart. I explained that the emergency services would want to help them, just like I did.

> I hope that in the future, gentleness will be recognized and valued much more. We rarely celebrate someone's gentleness. It is precious, it is powerful and it can undoubtedly help save lives.

15

SUPPORTING SOMEONE THROUGH MORE THAN ONE CRISIS

You may be supporting someone who has experienced a suicidal crisis before – perhaps several times. There are many reasons why this can happen. It may be that they have an underlying mental health condition. They may have repeated depressive episodes, for example. This might be part of bipolar disorder, where someone has both depressive episodes (low mood) and manic or hypomanic episodes (high or elated mood).

If someone has *a history of trauma*, this can also cause them to have more than one suicidal crisis. Childhood trauma can have a long-term effect on someone's mental health, as can severe trauma in adulthood, when it is not treated.

So it's about looking for the *underlying reasons* why they are continuing to have episodes where they have suicidal thoughts.

WHEN THEY HAVEN'T HAD THE RIGHT HELP

It is possible that they have not been able to get the right professional help. They may have experienced severe trauma but are unable to access psychological therapy (including trauma-focused therapy). They may be experiencing overwhelming post-traumatic symptoms, but are not getting the help they need for those symptoms. They are not getting help to process the traumatic event.

Sometimes it's because *professionals have not yet fully understood them* and their individual needs. If clinicians haven't yet understood them properly, it can result in getting an incorrect diagnosis – or no diagnosis at all – or to not getting the particular treatment or care plan that would be helpful to them.

There are times when a family member may think that their loved one is showing signs of a particular diagnosis – but the professionals caring for them have diagnosed them with something else. In this situation, professionals will usually really value the family's input, and will be very grateful for the information that they can provide. It helps in their understanding of the person under their care. But sometimes, family members feel that their opinions or concerns about diagnosis or treatments are not being heard.

In this situation, it can help to know that *your loved one can ask for a second opinion*. They have the right to ask for a second opinion about diagnosis. They also have the right to ask for a second opinion about treatment. They can ask for either, or for both. So they may feel that they have the right diagnosis, but that their care plan is not working for them.

We have helped a number of clients to request second opinions. Sometimes it has led to a different course of treatment. For example, one of our clients was told by her psychiatric team that they didn't think that individual psychological therapy would help her. She felt very strongly that it would. She had experienced several suicidal crises and she felt that trauma was at the root of this. So she asked for a second opinion. The second opinion assessment was with a psychologist in a different psychiatric team. The result was that the assessing psychologist agreed with her that psychological therapy was appropriate, and shortly afterwards she started the therapy.

Sometimes we find that our clients have had one type of therapy already, but it hasn't helped them. For example, many people find dialectical behaviour therapy really beneficial, but one of our clients felt it hadn't been quite right for her, and that she needed something more. She had really struggled with the group therapy aspect of it. It had been hard for her to speak in a group situation. Clinicians in the psychological therapies service said they didn't think it would benefit her to have a different therapy. She asked for a second opinion, and this led to her being offered a different kind of therapy. Schema therapy and mentalization-based therapy are two examples of other therapies, which are being used increasingly.

In the UK, many NHS mental health services have Complex Psychological Therapies services which can offer several different kinds of treatments. In other countries, your doctor or physician can give advice on how to see a psychologist. Additionally, the relevant national psychological association can provide information on how to find a psychologist near you: the American Psychological Association, Canadian Psychological Association, British Psychological Society or Australian Psychological Society, for example. Their details are at the end of this book. In the USA, your local or state psychological association can also be a source of information.

THE EXPERT KNOWLEDGE OF FAMILY AND FRIENDS

The input and knowledge of family and friends is so vital. Family and friends see so much that doctors and psychiatrists don't, because they usually have knowledge of the person over many years. They have spent much more time with them and have a deeper relationship with them.

The reason I was diagnosed with bipolar disorder was because of a close friend. I had been in a deep depression for a period of time, but then went into a period where I was high, elated, full of energy and out every night. At first, he was just relieved that I was out of the depressive episode. But then he thought more about it, and said: "Do you think you might have bipolar disorder?" It had not occurred to me, despite the fact that there is a family history of bipolar disorder.

My doctor was very willing to listen to my friend's observations. They monitored my moods and referred me to a psychiatrist who was a specialist in mood disorders. This led to the bipolar disorder diagnosis.

> If you feel that clinicians are not listening to you, and your friend or loved one agrees, you can ask another organization to communicate and advocate for you.

At our Suicide Crisis Centre, we regularly communicate with psychiatric services to advocate for people who are struggling to be heard – or to access the services they need.

It's not just getting a different diagnosis or treatment that can help. Sometimes it's about professionals taking a different approach. It's about working with the person to find out how clinicians could create a different kind of care plan that is personally tailored to them. Psychiatric services are starting to focus more on a "person-centred approach", rather than just treating someone according to a diagnosis.

Alternatively, your friend or loved one may find that charities provide a different kind of service, which is better suited to their needs. We set up a suicide crisis centre to provide an alternative type of care for people who would be reluctant to use psychiatric services, and for people who had used psychiatric services but had struggled to engage or had found those services were not right for them.

As well as getting suitable professional help, many people find that they also develop their own personalized "care plan" eventually. I'll explain more about care plans in the next chapter.

IF YOUR FRIEND OR LOVED ONE MAKES A SUICIDE ATTEMPT

You may hear about the suicide attempt of a friend or family member directly from them. You may hear it from someone else. You may receive a phone call to tell you that your loved one is in hospital, for example.

The aftermath: The impact on you

Understandably, you are likely to be feeling intense and powerful emotions. You're likely to feel shocked, frightened and deeply distressed. You may even feel anger toward your loved one – this often originates from the shock and fear of coming so close to losing them. It's important not to express anger to your loved one, though, nor to chastise them. But it is so important that you can express these feelings, whether it's to a friend, family member, or a professional. This is a profoundly distressing event and you need to be supported, too.

How your friend or family member may be feeling

Your loved one may still be experiencing the same deep emotional pain which led them to attempt to end their life. They may be experiencing the same loss of hope, and feelings of worthlessness or of being a burden. On top of this, they may be experiencing acute physical pain, serious injuries or internal damage – the effects of the suicide attempt.

After a suicide attempt, someone may be experiencing physical chaos. For example, a substantial drugs overdose will affect the body for many days afterwards. This combination of physical chaos and emotional turmoil leaves them acutely vulnerable to making another suicide attempt in the days afterwards.

They may also be experiencing feelings of guilt about the impact on loved ones, friends and work colleagues. However, some survivors will feel disappointment, distress or anger that they are still alive. Some experience shock, confusion or disbelief that they are still alive. They may feel emotionally numb. Other survivors feel relief that they have survived. They may feel remorse about having attempted suicide.

What to do

There is a significant risk of another suicide attempt in the days afterwards. It's important to make sure that they have the right professional help in place. We know that it is really important that we support clients intensively at our Suicide Crisis Centres after they have made a suicide attempt. We are acutely aware of their increased risk.

What to ask

If someone you know tells you that they have made a suicide attempt:

- **Ask whether they have received medical help.** A medication overdose can have fatal consequences several days after taking it. The effects may not be apparent immediately – some drugs act slowly. Other suicide methods can also leave survivors with lasting physical effects and it's vital that they have medical attention.
- **Ask whether they are still feeling suicidal.** Chapter 7 gives guidance about this, and the right professionals to contact, depending on their current level of risk.

What to say

Tell them that you love them, that you are so glad that they have survived, that you are here for them and you want to help. You can tell them that you are so sorry for the pain they experienced that led them to want to end their life.

I know that survivors of suicide attempts in hospital sometimes say that the simple act of holding their hand provides a form of comfort, reassurance, security and safety that is hard to express in words. The physical pain of a suicide attempt can be so hard to endure, and physical comfort can help. Many people don't realize how powerful physical touch can be, and what it can convey to a person who is experiencing profound emotional or physical pain.

Find out what professional crisis help is in place for them. It's important to clarify who they can call in the night or in the early hours of the morning, if they feel that they want to end their life again at those times. It does not have to be you, but it is vital that there is someone (professional or someone they know) who they would feel able to contact. If they tell you that they won't contact anyone, let a doctor or professional know this.

When they are ready to talk about it, you can try to explore what led to the attempt and what the particular triggers were. Try to find out if there were barriers to seeking help. They may have tried to contact crisis services but no one replied. You can help them to save additional numbers in their phone so they have several alternatives.

Ask them if they want other people to know about their suicide attempt and if so, who. If they are willing for other friends or family members to be informed, it can bring additional support. They can be part of the supportive "team" who can check in with them, and let them know how much they mean to everyone.

Talk about making a safety plan with them. Even if they reject this idea and feel uncomfortable with the idea of actually making a safety plan, you can still try to explore many of the topics that are in a safety plan with them: personal triggers, who they can call, and what is helpful to them when they are feeling suicidal, as well as personal strategies which help them stay safe. I'll explain more about what is in a safety plan in the next chapter.

16

HELPING SOMEONE TO CREATE THEIR OWN CARE PLAN AND SAFETY PLAN

One of the most helpful aspects of being diagnosed with bipolar disorder was that it made me realize that I was going to have more depressive episodes in the future. It helped me to prepare for them. I knew that I could go into very deep depressions, and so I started to look at things I could do to try to help prevent that from happening. I planned ahead for my next depressive episode, while I was mentally well between episodes.

Some of us find it really helpful to devise our own "care plan". You can help your friend or family member to create their own version of this, if they don't have one already.

It's important to emphasize that this is not *instead of* professional help, though. Having access to ongoing help and support is vital.

And although my own personal strategies have really helped me in depressive episodes, I know that I may still reach a point where my own strategies are not enough, and I need significant professional help myself.

CREATING A PERSONALIZED CARE PLAN

My plan was that I would draw on personal strategies, which could help prevent me from going into a deeper depression. As soon as I started to dip into depression, I would do things to help to stop myself from deteriorating further. The aim was to have a milder depressive episode – not one that was so deep that it might put my life at risk.

These are some of the things that have helped me, which your friend or family member could include in their plan:

Physical self-care

Physical self-care is an important part of my personal care plan in depressive episodes. This includes taking some exercise every day, such as walking.

Research has shown that exercise has anti-depressant effects. A study in 2018 focused on analyzing the impact of exercise (such as walking and jogging) on people who had been diagnosed with clinical depression.[20] The research showed that aerobic exercise had "large" or "moderate to large" anti-depressant effects.

Eating well

Eating well is important, too. As well as having meals that are healthy, it's good to also include *foods that your friend or loved one associates with comfort.*

Missing meals – and a lack of food – can really have a very detrimental effect on someone's mood and mental health.

We regularly find that clients at our Suicide Crisis Centre have not eaten, sometimes for days. But they will often accept the food we offer them. So your friend or loved one may feel able to eat, with your gentle encouragement – or if you offer them food or cook them something. As I've said before, food can be very symbolic of care and love.

Staying connected with friends and family

If they are finding it hard to talk on the phone or to be with people, then other forms of communication, especially written communication, become more important: text messaging, emails and social media contact, for example.

Spending time in nature

Spending as much time as possible in nature can also be an important part of the care plan. Many of us feel very at home in nature. We notice the beauty in nature and focus on the detail of the landscape around us. It can be a multi-sensory experience. We can listen to the sounds of nature, especially birdsong. Some of us use touch, too. For example, touching or leaning against a tree (and feeling its solidity) can be grounding and calming. It can also give a sense of connection with nature. We can also connect with wild animals or farm animals as we walk through fields.

Research has shown that spending time in nature has positive benefits for people who are depressed.[21] And one study in the USA, which focused on college-aged students, found that as little as ten minutes sitting or walking in a natural setting had positive benefits for the students' mental health.[22]

Creative activities

Creative activities such as art and writing also help many of us. Even when depression starts to cloud my thinking and robs me of my energy, I still try to write a little. But if writing feels too much then there are alternatives, such as colouring in pictures. The person you are concerned about can create beautiful things for family and friends. Deciding to colour a picture (or create something else) so that they can give or send it to a friend can make the activity even more meaningful.

Activities or things that comfort them or connect them with a safe and happy past

Some people find this helpful. It can include watching familiar television programmes that remind them of childhood or early adulthood and time spent with family and friends. For me, it's the sitcom *Friends*. It has positive associations with a safe and happy past spent with family and friends. One of my friends is aware of this and he watches the programme at the same time as me, in his own home, many miles away. The repeats are still on various television channels. This is a clever way of staying connected with me, through this shared activity, at a time when I am finding it hard to be with people.

Some of our clients have instinctively found their own ways of feeling comforted, or of feeling connected to a safe past.

One of our clients found that he was collecting military items, including a military jacket that he liked to keep beside him when he was at home. He bought all the items from various websites. One of the most influential people in his childhood had been a family friend who was in the military. He'd had a difficult childhood but this man had been kind, caring and had devoted a lot of time to him. He had never forgotten him. Keeping a military jacket beside him brought him comfort and peace and connected him to someone who was a source of love and kindness.

Activities which connect them with animals

There is a lot of research about how animals affect our mental health positively – and we don't need to have pets to get the positive effects.

Recent research in the UK has shown that watching birds in the garden and in the local neighbourhood has beneficial effects for our mental health.[23]

Placing bird feeders near the window can bring an array of different visiting birds. I have a robin who visits daily now, and I love the sense of connection I feel to him. Several of our clients have commented on how the regular visits of birds are comforting to them, too.

COMFORT IN ANIMALS

We know that pets – or "companion animals" – have a very positive impact on people who are experiencing mental health difficulties. Recent research in England has highlighted the strong sense of "connectivity" between pets and humans, and the contribution pets make to "emotional support in times of crises" together with "their ability to help manage symptoms when they arise".[24]

Although I don't have a pet, I have found ways to connect with dogs and cats. They often come up to greet me when I am out on a walk. This happens almost every time I walk outside now, probably because I find myself making eye contact with them. I love the connection and communication with them. I love how dogs often see an approaching human as a potential new friend, and rush up to say hello. Their affectionate, enthusiastic greeting can be so disarming. Their optimism, enthusiasm, zest for life and their unconditional love for all humans are a source of pleasure to me.

If you have a pet, it may help your friend or family member to spend time with them.

Even watching cats and dogs on social media can have a really positive effect – or watching animal programmes on television or on animal websites. I know many people find this therapeutic. Sometimes the social media videos are funny, sometimes they are simply adorable, but they bring great comfort.

As I have mentioned before, it can be easier for some people to connect with animals than with people. In particular, this can be the case when someone finds it hard to trust people because of past traumatic events.

And not everyone feels able to talk. That is why the sense of feeling connected to animals can be so important. We can communicate with animals in a different way – through touch and eye contact, for example. I know that many of our clients take comfort from just being near a family member's pet or a neighbour's pet – sitting beside them on the sofa, for example, or feeling their neighbour's dog pressed up against their feet as it sleeps.

It's why some people find therapy with horses (equine therapy) so helpful. Several of our clients who have experienced trauma have found this transformative. They have formed deep and lasting connections with horses.

Lights

Lights can bring comfort and reassurance, as well as being a source of beauty. There is probably a symbolic aspect to this, too: finding light among the darkness. Whether it is solar lights in the garden or twinkly fairy lights on the windowsill, it can all help. I now have a garden full of different solar lights decorating the trees and plants. This helps me in winter, too. It gets dark so early, and these lights create a landscape of beauty and light, which I can see from my window.

Making the home into a safe haven

Some of us find that there's a seasonal aspect to our depressive episodes. Some people are more vulnerable to depression in autumn and spring. Others find the winter difficult and start to feel lower in mood when the summer ends, because they are anticipating winter.

> It can help to make the home into a safe haven, when autumn arrives, to try to help counteract any negative associations that winter brings. I like to think of it as "cocooning".

A friend or family member can fill the room with things that feel comforting and cosy, and things which appeal to the different senses. For some people, that includes fluffy soft blankets and cushions (touch), twinkly lights and flowering plants (visual comfort), lavender essential oils (smell) and soft music or other comforting sounds like recordings of birdsong (sound). Wearing comfortable pyjamas and wrapping ourselves in a snuggly soft bathrobe or dressing gown can add to the feeling of safety and comfort.

CREATING A SAFETY PLAN

Some people also find it helpful to create a safety plan, and indeed the Royal College of Psychiatrists recommends using them. You can help your friend or family member to devise their own personalized safety plan.

The *personalized care plan* is for times when someone's mental health is starting to deteriorate.

The *safety plan* is for times when someone is having suicidal thoughts or is in distress. Like the care plan, the idea is to create it when your friend or family member is well, or not in crisis. It's about preparing for possible future crises. They may want to complete this on their own, or jointly with you. The safety plan is full of strategies they can use to help keep themselves safe, when they are feeling that they want to end their life – and these are very personalized strategies, individually tailored to them.

Make sure that you both have a copy of the safety plan. You can also talk about sharing the safety plan with other people, if your friend or family member agrees. It will be so helpful for other family members and of course professionals.

However, in outlining that a safety plan can be extremely helpful, I would also mention that many people who have experienced more than one suicidal crisis emphasize that every crisis is different. When they are asked by clinicians, "What did you do last time you felt like this?" they may reply: "I haven't felt like this before. It's different this time." This is why professional help is so important. It's vital that the person doesn't feel that they are being asked to use their own personal strategies instead of professional help. *If they are saying that the strategies they have used before are not helping, then it is really important that we all hear this – including professionals.*

What should a safety plan contain?

A safety plan will usually include things like:

Triggers: Are there specific things or events which have triggered suicidal thoughts in the past? If so, you or they can note these down so that you are aware of the potential risk, if similar circumstances happen again. For example, triggers might include specific times of the year (such as significant anniversaries – including the anniversary of traumatic events or birthdays of family members who have died). Triggering events may include things like relationship difficulties with their partner, or the ending of a relationship. For other people, reminders of a painful or traumatic event may be a trigger: certain images and smells can take them back to the event. They may feel that they are re-living it. Some people are more vulnerable when there are changes in their professional care, for example the ending of psychological therapy or a change of psychiatrists, or when they have a change of support worker, particularly if they have built a strong and trusting relationship with them. But it's important to be aware that there may not be an obvious trigger for everyone, or *there may be a different trigger every time they have a suicidal crisis.*

Warning signs: Are there warning signs that indicate that their mental health is deteriorating – for example, changes in mood, thoughts and behaviour? They may start to show increased levels of anger or they may start to have paranoid thoughts, for example. Or they may start to withdraw from family and friends. They might stop communicating with people.

Helpful personal strategies: This could include some of the strategies from the personalized care plan, or from previous chapters in this book, such as grounding techniques. It can include things that soothe and comfort them.

Reasons to stay alive: Write all of these down in the safety plan, too. For ideas of the kind of things to include, see pages 133-138.

People who can help and support them: Who do they find it helpful and supportive to be with, during times of crisis or distress?

What friends and family can do to help: How can friends and family best support them – what can they do that is helpful? The safety plan can be very individual and can include messages from family and friends.

Reducing the immediate risk: What items might need to be removed, to reduce the risk of harm?

Safe place: Include a list of places where they can go to feel safer. That may be the home of a friend or family member, or it may be a crisis centre or Emergency Department. Alternatively, they may have a safe place in a particular part of their own home.

Professional help: What kind of professional help is supportive for them when they are having suicidal thoughts? What is it important for professionals to know about them? What kinds of things are helpful?

Professional contacts: the professionals and organizations that they can contact, with phone numbers. *Make sure that the numbers are saved on their phone, too.*

What do they find unhelpful when they are in distress or having suicidal thoughts? This may be things that professionals or friends and family members have said or done in the past, when they have been in crisis or distressed.

It can be helpful for your friend or family member to keep messages from significant people in a box or other container. These messages from friends and family can be specifically written for them to read in times of crisis, or they can be loving messages that they have received in the past. The messages or letters often contain words that remind the person that they are loved and cared about – and describe their unique individual qualities, and the difference they make. The box could contain photos, too. It could also include any messages of thanks or any positive feedback they have received from people they have helped at work or in their voluntary work – reminding them of the difference they make.

The messages or letters could be written by professionals, if someone is more isolated. I remember how I sent cards to one of our clients who lived alone, at a time when he felt very isolated. He told me that he used to read what I had written when he started to feel more vulnerable and alone. He said that it reminded him that we cared about him, and it helped him to hold us in his mind.

Even if your friend or family member says that they are not comfortable with the idea of a safety plan, it can be helpful to talk with them about the different aspects of it. It can help you to understand more about what is likely to be helpful (and unhelpful) to them during a period of crisis.

17

LOOKING AFTER YOURSELF

Supporting a friend or family member through a suicidal crisis is one of the most giving and rewarding things you can do. But in caring for them, it is so important that you also care for yourself, and have access to support.

In the course of my work, I have met many of the family members and friends of clients who we are supporting at our Suicide Crisis Centres. When they explain what helps their own wellbeing during this period, they often mention:

- having someone who provides *emotional support* for them as the "caregiver"
- having access to *peer support* – contact with other people who are supporting someone in mental health crisis
- having *periods of time when they can rest* and do things that are therapeutic and positive for their own mental health and wellbeing
- their own *personal strategies and self-care*
- the involvement of *other family members or friends*

- knowing that their family member or friend *has relevant professional support*
- having *someone they can turn to for advice* about what to do in different situations as they arise

EMOTIONAL SUPPORT

For some people, the emotional support is provided by other family members or friends. Being able to talk things through with someone else can help enormously. It is important to be able to ventilate your own feelings.

But most people I have met also said that they needed access to a professional for support, too. Sometimes there are things they didn't feel able to say to another friend or family member.

Some people talk to their doctor, who can also refer them for other professional support or counselling.

I have spoken to many parents and they have shared their experiences of supporting a loved one through suicidal crisis. Some of them have been kind enough to write to me, too. One parent described how she and her husband cared for their daughter during the early stages of a period of mental health crisis:

"We were just on automatic pilot, coping as best we could, hour by hour, day by day. We did not have time to think about our own care; we simply lived and breathed caring, keeping our loved one safe. The strange thing is that we did not even consider ourselves to be carers, or even recognize the word. No one suggested we were carers. We did not know where to go for help – so we received none."

She explained that eventually, someone from the mental health crisis team told her about the local carers' centre: "The carers' centre had existed for nearly 25 years, but we had no knowledge of it. That was the beginning of a journey that helped us get some support."

YOUR ROLE AS A CARER

Recognizing that you are a carer can be the start of getting more help. Many of us don't realize that we are, until someone tells us. As well as local carers' centres, many countries have national charities such as Carers UK, Family Carers Ireland, the National Alliance for Caregiving in the USA and Carers Australia. Some of these organizations can provide advice and support to carers (also known as "caregivers" in some countries). Some of them provide access to counselling and also support groups where you can meet other carers. Many of these support groups are specifically for people caring for someone with a mental health condition.

I have been invited to visit mental health carers' groups in different parts of the UK, and they sometimes tell me how hard it can be to access one-to-one professional support and help for themselves. There is a need for more to be done to support the wellbeing and mental health of carers.

One mother described how valuable it had been to call a national helpline at a time when she had no access to other professional support, while she was caring for her daughter during a period of prolonged mental health crisis: "I recall that I made two calls to the helpline and just cried continuously for an hour each time. The kindness of the call operator, just listening to me while I cried, helped so much."

PEER SUPPORT

Many people who are caring for a family member or friend who is going through a period of mental health crisis have found it extremely helpful to talk to other people who are in a similar situation. They say it has so many benefits. It is often in local carer support groups that they find this peer support.

They explain that talking to other people in similar circumstances means that they no longer feel alone in this situation; they can be with people who immediately understand. Other carers have often had similar experiences, commenting: "It was the camaraderie of other carers – who understood the pain I felt for my loved one – who helped me the most." One parent explained that it could be hard to talk to other friends about "something so private – my daughter's mental health crisis".

Importantly, many carers explain that they can say things to other caregivers that they would not feel able to say to their friends or even to professionals. "I know that other carers won't judge me." "I can be really honest and say things that I wouldn't feel able to say to friends."

Some local carer organizations have organized "carer to carer" schemes, a father explained to me. Not everyone can attend organized carer support group meetings, and so these alternative schemes offer one-to-one peer support. He explained: "Volunteers who were (or had been) carers were matched to a carer who was in need of support. Some carers wanted a close match, for example someone caring for a family member with a similar diagnosis. Support was provided by phone, face-to-face meetings or email, depending on the wishes of the carer and volunteer. The matching was for about an hour a week for six months. Volunteers were trained and had several roles: listening, supporting, sharing experiences, signposting and chatting. It was not counselling, and if it became clear that there was a need for this, then volunteers would signpost the carer to relevant help."

He also explained how he set up an alternative support network that helped him: "You can establish reciprocal '24/7 personal friends or family'. It does not matter what time a 24/7 friend calls, you just listen to them. I personally have several 24/7 friends. Calls are rare but very precious."

PERSONAL STRATEGIES FOR REST AND SELF-CARE

Having periods of time to rest is very important. A man who was caring for his partner who was in mental health crisis explained that it was often about creating "moments of self-care".

He said: "A warm bath, something good to eat and some time outside with nature are all invaluable. Listening to music can be a good release, too. Reading, gardening and walking help me. Writing can be a great outlet and help take me away from internalizing the experiences I have had. I have also tried 'mindful photography,' and can vouch for the value of being helped to appreciate the beauty in simple things."

Another caregiver pointed out: "Remember that your mental and physical health is just as important as that of the person you are caring for."

Some caregivers said they felt guilty if they took time for self-care, but it is so important. One carer said: "If you do not take breaks, you will eventually have to take a much longer break, because we all have a limit. There's a risk that you will become unwell yourself, if you don't take care of your own mental health."

> By looking after your own wellbeing, you are indirectly helping your friend or family member. It is much harder to care for someone when you are exhausted and stressed.

You can also do shared activities with your friend or family member that are beneficial to both of you – activities that are therapeutic or which allow the mind to rest. These include things like walking in nature, gardening or watching a film together. A mother explained that she found it therapeutic to "walk mindfully while accompanying my daughter, when she felt able to leave the house".

She explained that she also took comfort from "stroking our dog. He could sense the anguish in our home and did his best to bring comfort." Like other carers, she described "moments of self-care": "Looking up at the clouds whenever I walked into the garden to hang out washing to dry. That was 'my time'. And listening to the buzzing of bees in the garden – if you focus enough, you block out everything else around you in that moment."

She added that she found relief in "crying – often. It's important to let the emotions flow. Bottling things up can affect your mental and physical health."

She added, poignantly: "Never let go of hope; that word in itself made the situation bearable. It was all we had most of the time and it allowed us to cling on to the prospect of positive change." Now, many months later, she describes how her daughter is "able to embrace life again".

INVOLVING OTHER FAMILY MEMBERS AND FRIENDS

By involving other family members or friends, you can share the caring role with others. It allows time for you to rest and recover, while someone else is spending time with your family member or friend. It also means that you can get their opinion and viewpoints at times when you are not sure what is best to do for the person in crisis.

One of our clients explained: "My friend Rob took me walking and talking. My cousin Jane comforted me. She had known me for most of my life and I could trust her and open up to her. She knew I needed professional help, too, and she used to take me to the Suicide Crisis Centre and collect me afterwards. Jane and the team at the Suicide Crisis Centre had a joint quest to ensure I survived."

GETTING THE RIGHT SUPPORT FOR YOUR LOVED ONE

One of the biggest triggers for stress among caregivers is when a loved one isn't able to get the mental health care that they are seeking. It can create intense anxiety, concern and fear for their loved one's wellbeing.

In Chapter 15, I explained some of the ways you can help someone who is struggling to get the right care and treatment. Usually, mental health services and clinical services are very aware of the importance of working closely with family and friends of the person in crisis. But it can cause huge stress if you feel that professionals are not listening to your concerns about your family member or friend. Understandably, patient confidentiality often means that doctors and clinicians are not able to share information with you, without the patient's consent. But this does not mean that doctors and clinicians cannot *receive* information from you. Indeed, they should be very willing to listen to any concerns or information that you share about a patient. By sharing, you are helping clinicians to provide the best and safest care for their patient.

The General Medical Council has given specific guidance to doctors in the UK about this. In its ethical guidance for doctors, it explains: "If someone close to the patient wants to discuss their concerns about the patient's health without involving the patient, you should not refuse to listen to their views or concerns on the grounds of confidentiality. The information they give you might be helpful in your care of the patient."[25] The same guiding principle should apply to other clinicians, too. Most doctors and clinicians positively welcome information from family and friends, of course, and are thankful for it.

If you are concerned about a loved one's deteriorating mental health and you feel that clinicians are not hearing you, you can ask to talk to someone higher up. This is usually a clinical manager or a clinical director, if your loved one is under mental health services. You can explain that you need to talk to them that same day. But if it's an urgent situation and their usual team or doctor doesn't seem to be responding, then you can use other routes to get immediate help for your loved one, including the Emergency Department or emergency services.

When you are trying to get the right care for someone over the longer term, then local carer or mental health charities or local advocacy services may be able to advocate for you and your loved one.

ACCESS TO ADVICE AND INFORMATION

Many family members have said it makes a real difference if there are professionals they can contact to get advice or information when different situations arise. Many of the national charities have helplines where they can give practical information about possible routes forward. These include carers' charities such as Carers UK and the National Alliance for Caregiving in the USA, mental health charities such as Mind and Rethink Mental Illness in the UK, and the National Alliance on Mental Illness (NAMI) in the USA.

As well as a telephone advice service, the charity Rethink Mental Illness offers over 200 different factsheets, on subjects including "Your rights to access treatment", "Second opinions", and "Confidentiality and information sharing – for carers, friends and family". They also have specialist leaflets, including factsheets that focus on specific situations, for example when someone goes into prison.

The National Alliance on Mental Illness provides a national helpline, which can offer support, listening and information, and they have a number of local family support groups (open to friends as well as family members of someone who has a mental health condition). The organization also provides resource guides, including a guidebook for mental health caregivers.

If your loved one is under a crisis service or under mental health services, you can talk to them, too. If they are under psychiatric services, their clinicians may be able to give you specific advice. Increasingly, psychiatric services talk in terms of "working in partnership" with families and close friends of their patients. Charities providing crisis services are usually very willing to talk to you and help, too.

While you are doing such wonderful work in supporting your friend, colleague or family member, you are equally precious. Caring for them often places huge demands on you at times, even though you give this care willingly and gladly. Your own mental and physical health is equally important, and I hope that some of the strategies and information in this chapter will help you maintain it.

18

PROFESSIONAL HELP

As I have explained throughout the book, it's important that your friend or family member can access professional help, as well as the support and care you are giving them. This chapter explains about some of the different kinds of help available.

DOCTORS OR PHYSICIANS

Your friend or family member's doctor or physician can be a source of professional help throughout a period of crisis. They can also refer your friend/family member to psychiatric services or other crisis services. However, in some areas people can refer themselves to mental health crisis services.

Later on, as they start to recover from their suicidal crisis, the doctor can refer them for ongoing help such as counselling, which can help with some of the underlying factors that have contributed to their crisis, such as bereavement or trauma. The doctor can also refer them to other specialist services.

MENTAL HEALTH SERVICES (PSYCHIATRIC SERVICES)

Mental health services often have a number of specialist teams, which involve different professionals including psychiatrists and psychiatric nurses. In the UK, most psychiatric services also have teams of psychologists. In the USA and other countries, you can ask your family doctor or physician about the most appropriate route to see a psychiatrist or psychologist.

Psychiatrists are specialist doctors who have already gone through several years of general medical training before specializing in psychiatry. They can diagnose different psychiatric conditions and prescribe medication, and they often take the lead in decisions about someone's care plan.

Psychologists provide different psychological therapies (also known as talking therapies). Some of the therapies they can provide include cognitive behavioural therapy (CBT), dialectical behaviour therapy (DBT) and mentalization-based therapy (MBT).

National Institute for Health and Care Excellence (NICE) clinical guidance states that DBT can be particularly helpful for helping people looking to manage self-harm.[26]

The NICE clinical guidance for post-traumatic stress disorder cites trauma-focused CBT and eye movement desensitization and reprocessing (EMDR) as treatments.[27]

There are several other types of therapy, too. Even if someone has already had one type of therapy in the past, it is possible to have a different kind.

Psychological therapy is usually started when someone is feeling more stable and when the period of crisis has ended. It can help someone to process the underlying reasons (such as past trauma), which may have contributed to their suicidal crisis.

CRISIS TEAMS
(WITHIN PSYCHIATRIC SERVICES)

In the UK, most psychiatric services that are provided by the National Health Service (NHS) have crisis teams working in the community. These were set up as an alternative to psychiatric hospitals, because some people find it more helpful and less restrictive to be supported in their own home. Crisis teams can support people intensively during a mental health crisis. In some areas, people can self-refer, but in other areas it needs a GP referral or a referral from another medical or psychiatric professional.

There are also psychiatric hospitals where patients can be admitted for a period of time. In the UK, patients are either admitted as "informal" (voluntary) patients or "formal" patients (detained under the Mental Health Act or "sectioned").[19] In the USA, Australia and some other countries they use the term "involuntary admission" or "involuntary psychiatric hospitalization" rather than "sectioning".

In the UK, most people who experience a suicidal crisis won't be detained under the Mental Health Act – nor even admitted voluntarily to psychiatric hospital – it is much more likely that they will receive support in the community from crisis teams. Many other countries have community-based mental health care and treatment options, too.

EMERGENCY HELP

When someone is at immediate risk of suicide, or severely mentally unwell, contact your country's emergency services. These include:

UK: 999
USA and Canada: 911
Australia: 000
New Zealand: 111

EMERGENCY DEPARTMENT

You can also take your friend or family member to the Emergency Department at the local general hospital, if they are at immediate risk of suicide. In the UK, there are psychiatric teams based in the general hospitals and this means that they are on site and able to assess people who come into the Emergency Department.

As well as psychiatric and medical services, there are charities and organizations that provide services.

CRISIS SERVICES RUN BY CHARITIES

Some countries have additional crisis services, which are run by charities or other organizations. These have emerged as an alternative to psychiatric crisis services because there was a realization that some people would benefit from a different type of care.

Our Suicide Crisis Centre opened in 2013, a year after our charity (Suicide Crisis) was created.

NATIONAL TELEPHONE HELPLINES

There are national suicide prevention helplines in many countries, and these provide excellent support in times of crisis.

UK and Ireland: The Samaritans on 116 123

USA: National Suicide Prevention Lifeline on 1-800-273-8255. From 2022 this will change to a three-digit number – you will simply call 988. It will be much easier for people to remember just three numbers.

Canada: Canada Suicide Prevention Helpline on 1-833-456-4560. There are plans to change this to a three-digit number: 988.

Australia: Lifeline on 13 11 14

New Zealand: "Need to talk?" on 1737

EPILOGUE

Thoughts on Why Clients Survive at Our
Suicide Crisis Centres

I thought it might be helpful to end the book with some reflections about our Suicide Crisis Centres. Currently, we only provide a suicide crisis service in Gloucestershire in the UK, but we are contacted by people from other parts of the country (and indeed in other parts of the world) who wish to learn more about how we work, or who wish to have a suicide crisis centre in their region or country, and would like advice about how to make that happen. We are always keen to try to help.

We are often asked the question: "Why do all your clients survive?" I think it is because of a combination of factors, which include:

- the model of service
- our approach and ethos
- methods we use

Our first Suicide Crisis Centre was opened in 2013, and the second was opened a few years later.

THE MODEL OF SERVICE: HOW WE OPERATE

We provide a combination of suicide crisis centre and home visits, and emergency phone lines. This means that we have more ways to keep connected with our clients, and our ability to travel to clients' homes means we can get to them quickly in an emergency. We recognize that if someone is at immediate risk of suicide, they may be too distressed to come to our crisis centre, so we need to go to them.

FREQUENCY OF CONTACT

We are in daily contact with most of our clients during the period of intense crisis. This is usually daily face-to-face contact, but we may use additional forms of contact, too. We might need to use additional phone, text or email contact as well as the appointments. This gradually becomes less frequent as they start to come out of crisis.

THE STRONG RELATIONSHIPS AND CONNECTIONS WE BUILD WITH OUR CLIENTS

We care very much about our clients. We rarely need to tell them this. It is often they who tell us: "We know that you care." Our actions, as much as our words, show them this. We do everything we can to try to help them to survive.

Building a strong relationship of trust, connection and care is so vital. *If the quality of the relationship is good, it can sustain the person even when you are absent.* We see most of our clients for an hour a day when they are in crisis. This means that for 23 hours of the day, we are not with them. But the strong connection that we have built "holds" them and sustains them. They feel connected to us. And they know they can immediately contact us, if they need to. We are there for them the whole time.

One of our clients said it was like he carried us "in his pocket". It was a powerful metaphor, which explained the connection he felt with our team. It was like we were always with him. He said it gave him a sense of security to know that he could reach for us at any time – taking us out of his pocket for immediate help. When he eventually left our service, he sent us this message:

"You remain in my pocket for life – supporting, guiding and aiding my recovery."

He describes how the connection and care continues to sustain him, even after he has left our service.

His description of our services inspired the title of this book.

INDIVIDUALIZED CARE

We use a person-centred approach. We get to know our clients so that we can understand their individual needs. This means that we can provide care that is individually tailored to them.

BEING PROACTIVE AND TENACIOUS

Some statutory services and charities talk about "respecting a person's right" to end their life, if they are assessed as having the mental capacity to make that decision.[28] However, we take a different approach. When someone is at the point of suicide, they are almost always thinking in a very different way from usual. High levels of distress or mental illness (including depression) are influencing their thinking. For that reason, *we always intervene to protect the life of every client under our care.*

We are proactive about keeping in contact with our clients.

From the start, our approach has been that we would do everything we could to help each individual to survive.

BALANCING PROTECTING CLIENTS WITH GIVING THEM CONTROL

Feeling in control can be extremely important for many people, particularly if they have endured traumatic events where they have experienced a loss of control and felt powerless. Men have told us that they find being in control helpful, too. When they seek help and disclose deep and painful emotions for the first time, they can feel very vulnerable. It is as if they have taken off their protective armour. That can be a very uncomfortable feeling. But if we explain that *they are in control of their care,* it helps to counteract the feeling of vulnerability. They usually decide how often they see us and the kind of care they will receive... and they usually decide when they feel ready to leave us.

Although we put clients in control of their care as much as we can, we make sure that they are protected the whole of the time that they are under our services. They are wrapped in the safety net that we place around them. We actively intervene to protect their life. And although they usually decide how often they see us, there are times when we need to negotiate this with them, because we are concerned about them. We may feel it's important for us to see them more often than they suggest.

Some clients want to place more of the control in our hands, especially in the early stages. They may be experiencing shock, inner turmoil and deep distress and it may be hard for them to make any decisions about their care. A male client explained this in an email to us after he left our care:

"In those early days, in the depths of my crisis, I looked for your guidance to steer me out of the darkness.

My traumatic experience left me feeling blind and unable to move forward without you taking my hand, steadying me and leading me forward.

Then, eventually, I felt able to let go and walk beside you. Finally, you enabled me to walk on ahead of you toward recovery."

He explains so beautifully the gentle transition from being held, guided and supported, to gradually feeling able to take steps forward himself.

LIVED EXPERIENCE

Lived experience is at the heart of our work. I experienced suicidal crisis myself in 2012, and found the available services didn't work for me. That was why I felt that there was a need for something different: a suicide crisis centre with a different approach and ethos.

My lived experience means that *I understand what it is like to be at the point of suicide*, and to have attempted suicide.

Although my professional training is vital, my lived experience gives me knowledge and understanding that goes beyond that.

The lived experience of our first few clients further influenced our way of working.

Lived experience is embedded into our work and it affects how we work every day.

FLEXIBLE WAYS TO ACCESS OUR SERVICE AT THE START

Although most clients make contact with us by phone initially, some men say they would not have felt able to do this. They needed to make their first contact by text or email. This felt like a more comfortable first step than walking into a crisis centre or picking up a phone. Taking small steps can be helpful. They often send a very short message at first to see what kind of response they get – and how that feels.

The text or email contact continues for a few days. Through these messages, they start to build a connection and build trust with us. Then they feel ready to come in and see us.

Texting or emailing first also allows them to say things in writing that might be hard for them to say face-to-face.

We understand that some new clients need to start their journey with us gently and in small steps. We need to let them gradually build trust and connect with us at their own pace, and in the way that is comfortable for them. *It is important that we adapt to them, and that we do not expect them to adapt to a pace that is set by us.*

HIGHLY SKILLED TEAM

All except one of our team members are fully qualified counsellors. Many of the skills we learn in counselling training are so helpful when supporting people in crisis, as I explained in Chapter 8. Our team members have additional external training in suicide intervention skills. Further training was provided and arranged by our advising psychiatrist and other clinicians at the start. This related in particular to assessing suicide risk. We wanted to make sure that our suicide risk assessing was as rigorous as that of psychiatric clinicians.

But the personal qualities of our team members are just as important – they are kind, caring, empathic, sensitive, understanding and respectful. Their professional skills and personal qualities are of equal importance.

SMALL TEAM

Usually, only two members of our team support each client. This allows us to get to know clients well. It helps in building trust, and providing continuity of care.

Men in particular often tell us that they want to be supported by a very small team when they are in crisis. Some men under our care only feel able to be supported by one team member – the person who first assesses them. When they come to see us, they take the hugely courageous step of expressing their deep emotional pain, their distress and their fears. This may be something that they have never revealed to anyone before. It can be so hard for them to disclose this. They may only feel able to do so once. As such, they may feel able to show this level of vulnerability to only one person. Over time, they are usually willing to let us involve another member of our team. But it is the beginning that is so hard for them, and we recognize that.

OUR TEAM'S ABILITY TO ASSESS RISK ACCURATELY

Of course our ability to assess risk accurately is a significant part of why all our clients have survived. Clients who are assessed as being at high risk of suicide receive additional support. They have access to support 24 hours a day.

THE CONCEPT OF "ZERO SUICIDE"

We didn't originally set out to achieve zero suicide. We never set this as a goal or an ambition.

When we started to provide services, professionals from other services told me: "You must prepare yourself for the fact that people will take their own life." The prospect of clients dying was so painful that I replied, "I am going to do everything I can to try to prevent that from happening."

My approach was simply that *we would do everything that we could for each individual, to help them to survive.* That has been the strategy since the first day. It is what we continue to do, every day. It doesn't put us under pressure. It has felt entirely natural to do this from the start – a natural consequence of caring about our clients.

Ultimately, we have the same goal as services that adopt a zero suicide ambition.

As professionals, we need to be tenacious in helping people to survive suicidal crisis. I always believe that every client who comes to us can survive.

So when I am asked why all clients under our care have survived up to this date, I sometimes say: "I think it is about a combination of factors, which have all come together at this time and in this place."

But I think the most fundamental factor in all of it, is the relationship and strong connection that we build with our clients – the fact that we care about them, and care very much that they survive. This is something that can be replicated in psychiatric services and crisis services everywhere. And it is something that *you* already have in abundance, ready to give to your friend or family member, so you have a major advantage at the start of your journey with them through a suicidal crisis.

Thank you for everything you are giving to them. Thank you for your care, support and love through this painful journey.

ACKNOWLEDGEMENTS

I am so grateful to all the clients we have supported at our crisis centres. We have learned, and continue to learn, so much from you. Each of your experiences is unique, and each of you adds to our learning.

The last eight years would not have been possible without my exceptional colleagues at Suicide Crisis, and that includes our wonderful team who work with clients in crisis, our supportive trustees and our skilled advising psychiatrist and other advising clinicians.

Thank you so much to Tim, who works in our communications department at Suicide Crisis. Tim helps to edit all the charity's publications – and makes editing more fun than it should be. He is also a dear and supportive friend.

Thank you to the carers who contributed to Chapter 17, which focuses on how carers can look after their own wellbeing. Thank you for giving me permission to quote you. Your contributions have provided powerful testimonies and invaluable advice for readers.

My thanks also to Beth, Jo and the team at Welbeck Balance. The idea for the book was yours, and it is a book which mattered very much to you all to publish.

Special thanks and love to my wonderful parents, who I miss so much. They didn't live to see me set up the charity or the

Suicide Crisis Centres, but I feel that they have been alongside me. They gave me the best possible start in life, with their love and support, and they instilled values that I have carried with me. They also read all the "books" I wrote when I was a small child, and encouraged me to write more. Thank you also to my uncle Bill who was so supportive, and who demonstrated by example that individuality and following your own path in life is something to be cherished.

FURTHER HELP AND RESOURCES

SUICIDE CRISIS

For more information about the charity Suicide Crisis, visit suicidecrisis.co.uk or write to Suicide Crisis, P.O. Box 1344, Cheltenham, GL50 9FP, UK.

Suicide Crisis only provides a crisis service for Gloucestershire in the UK currently, but their team is actively working with other regions to help similar services to be created.

Other organizations, which offer help, support or information, including those named in the book are below.

NATIONAL TELEPHONE HELPLINES

Crisis Text Line (USA, Canada, Ireland, UK): www.crisistextline.org
   UK and Ireland: The Samaritans on 116 123
   USA: National Suicide Prevention Lifeline on 1-800-273-8255. From 2022, it will change to a three-digit number – you will simply call 988.
   Canada: Canada Suicide Prevention Helpline on 1-833-456-4560. There are plans to change this to a three-digit number: 988.
   Australia: Lifeline on 13 11 14
   New Zealand: "Need to talk?" on 1737

SUICIDE PREVENTION ORGANIZATIONS

UK
Campaign Against Living Miserably (CALM):
www.thecalmzone.net
PAPYRUS (dedicated to the prevention of young suicide):
www.papyrus-uk.org
The Samaritans: www.samaritans.org; helpline: 116 123
Support After Suicide Partnership:
supportaftersuicide.org.uk
Survivors of Bereavement by Suicide: uksobs.org

USA
American Foundation for Suicide Prevention: afsp.org
National Suicide Prevention Lifeline:
suicidepreventionlifeline.org
Jed Foundation (dedicated to the prevention of young
suicide): www.jedfoundation.org
Alliance of Hope for suicide loss survivors: allianceofhope.org

Canada
Canada Suicide Prevention Service:
www.crisisservicescanada.ca

Australia and New Zealand
Lifeline Australia: www.lifeline.org.au
Lifeline Aotearoa: www.lifeline.org.nz

GENERAL MENTAL HEALTH RESOURCES

UK
Heads Together: www.headstogether.org.uk
Hub of Hope: hubofhope.co.uk
Mental Health Foundation: www.mentalhealth.org.uk
Mind: www.mind.org.uk
Rethink Mental Illness: www.rethink.org
Samaritans: www.samaritans.org, helpline: 116 123
Scottish Association for Mental Health (SAMH):
www.samh.org.uk
Shout: www.giveusashout.org, text 85258
Young Minds: www.youngminds.org.uk

Europe
Mental Health Europe: www.mhe-sme.org
Mental Health Ireland: www.mentalhealthireland.ie

USA
Mentalhealth.gov: www.mentalhealth.gov
Mental Health America: www.mhanational.org
National Alliance on Mental Illness (NAMI): www.nami.org
National Institute of Mental Health: www.nimh.nih.gov

Canada
Canadian Mental Health Association: cmha.ca
eMentalHealth.ca: www.ementalhealth.ca

Australia and New Zealand

Beyond Blue: www.beyondblue.org.au

Head to Health: headtohealth.gov.au

Health Direct: www.healthdirect.gov.au

Mental Health Australia: mhaustralia.org

Mental Health Foundation of New Zealand:
www.mentalhealth.org.nz

SANE Australia: www.sane.org

SPECIFIC ISSUES HELP, SUPPORT AND INFORMATION

Autism

National Autistic Society (UK): www.autism.org.uk

Autism Society (USA): www.autism-society.org

Autism Awareness (Australia): www.autismawareness.com.au

Bullying

Bullying UK: www.bullying.co.uk

Stomp Out Bullying (USA): stompoutbullying.org

Bully Zero (Australia): www.bullyzero.org.au

Carers

Carers UK: www.carersuk.org

Family Carers Ireland: familycarers.ie

National Alliance for Caregiving (USA): caregiving.org

Carers Canada: carerscanada.ca
Carers Australia: carersaustralia.com.au
Carers New Zealand: carers.net.nz

LGBTQ+
LBGT Foundation (UK): lgbt.foundation
Trevor Project (USA): www.thetrevorproject.org
Q Life Counselling Service (Australia): qlife.org.au

PMDD
International Association for Premenstrual Disorders: iapmd.org

PSYCHOLOGICAL AND MEDICAL SOCIETIES AND ASSOCIATIONS

British Psychological Society (UK): bps.org.uk
Royal College of Psychiatrists (UK): rcpsych.ac.uk
American Psychological Association: apa.org
Canadian Psychological Association: cpa.ca
Australian Psychological Society: psychology.org.au
New Zealand Psychological Society: psychology.org.nz

REFERENCES

1. *Suicide*, World Health Organization (2019): www.who.int/news-room/fact-sheets/detail/suicide
2. *Suicide facts and figures: United States*, American Foundation for Suicide Prevention (2020): www.datocms-assets.com/12810/1587128056-usfactsfiguresflyer-2.pdf
3. *Suicides in England and Wales: 2019 Registrations*, Office for National Statistics (2020): www.ons.gov.uk/peoplepopulationandcommunity/birthsdeathsandmarriages/deaths/bulletins/suicidesintheunitedkingdom/2019registrations
4. *Depression in adults: recognition and management, Clinical Guideline CG90*, National Institute for Clinical Excellence (NICE) (2009): www.nice.org.uk/guidance/cg90/chapter/Key-priorities-for-implementation
5. *Psychosis information: for parents and carers*, Royal College of Psychiatrists (2020): www.rcpsych.ac.uk/mental-health/parents-and-young-people/information-for-parents-and-carers/psychosis-information-for-parents-and-carers
6. During our research into deaths by suicide in 2017-18, we attended inquests over a six-month period in Gloucestershire, UK. In 25 of the inquests, it was found that the deceased person had taken their own life. Our

full research report is a 44-page document. A shorter report of the headline findings is available on request from the charity Suicide Crisis: suicidecrisis.co.uk or write to Suicide Crisis, P.O. Box 1344, Cheltenham, GL50 9FP, UK.

7. *Impact of screening for risk of suicide: randomized controlled trial*, Crawford, Thana et al (2011), *British Journal of Psychiatry*, vol. 198,5: www.cambridge.org/core/journals/the-british-journal-of-psychiatry/article/impact-of-screening-for-risk-of-suicide-randomised-controlled-trial/C13EF2D1B4FC19F0867838D5D4106CDD

8. *Evaluating iatrogenic risk of youth suicide screening programs: A randomized controlled trial*, Gould, Marrocco, Kleinman et al (2005): jamanetwork.com/journals/jama/article-abstract/200641

9. *Suicide Act*, HM Government (1961): www.legislation.gov.uk/ukpga/Eliz2/9-10/60

10. Supreme Court Judgment in the case of R (Maughan) v HM Senior Coroner for Oxfordshire (2020): www.supremecourt.uk/cases/uksc-2019-0137.html

11. *Living alone, loneliness and lack of emotional support as predictors of suicide and self-harm: a nine-year follow up of the UK Biobank cohort*, Shaw, Cullen, Graham et al (2020): pubmed.ncbi.nlm.nih.gov/33096330/

12. *Self-harm and suicide in adults: final report of the Patient Safety Group*, Royal College of Psychiatrists (2020): www.rcpsych.ac.uk/docs/default-source/improving-care/better-

mh-policy/college-reports/college-report-cr229-self-harm-and-suicide.pdf

13. *Bereavement by suicide as a risk factor for suicide attempt: a cross-sectional national UK-wide study of 3432 young bereaved adults*, Pitman, Osborn, Randell et al (2016): bmjopen.bmj.com/content/6/1/e009948

14. *Dying from inequality. Socioeconomic disadvantage and suicidal behaviour summary report*, Samaritans (2017): media.samaritans.org/documents/Samaritans_Dying_from_inequality_report_-_summary.pdf

15. *Preventing prison suicide*, The Howard League for Penal Reform and the Centre for Mental Health (2016): howardleague.org/wp-content/uploads/2016/11/Preventing-prison-suicide-report.pdf

16. *Sexual identity, sex of sexual contacts, and health risk behaviors among students in grades 9-12: youth risk behavior surveillance, Atlanta, GA*, US Department of Health and Human Services (CDC, 2016): pubmed.ncbi.nlm.nih.gov/27513843/

17. *The report of the 2015 US transgender survey*, National Center for Transgender Equality, James SE, Herman JL, Rankin S, Keisling M, Mottet L, Anafi M (2016): www.ustranssurvey.org/reports

18. *Preventing suicide in England: third progress report of the cross-government outcomes strategy to save lives*, HM Government (2017): assets.publishing.service.gov.uk/government/uploads/system/uploads/attachment_data/file/582117/Suicide_report_2016_A.pdf

19. *Mental Health Act*, HM Government (1983): www.nhs.uk/mental-health/social-care-and-your-rights/mental-health-and-the-law/mental-health-act

20. *Aerobic exercise for adult patients with major depressive disorder in mental health services: a systematic review and meta-analysis*, Morres ID, Hatzigeorgiadis A, Stathi A et al (2018): pubmed.ncbi.nlm.nih.gov/30334597

21. *Interacting with nature improves cognition and affect for individuals with depression*, Berman, Marc G et al (2012), *Journal of Affective Disorders*, vol. 140,3: 300-5: www.sciencedirect.com/science/article/abs/pii/S0165032712002005

22. *Minimum time dose in nature to positively impact the mental health of college-aged students, and how to measure it: a scoping review*, Meredith GR, Rakow DA, Eldermire ERB, Madsen CG, Shelley SP, Sachs NA (2020), *Frontiers in Psychology 2020*, vol. 10: www.frontiersin.org/article/10.3389/fpsyg.2019.02942

23. *Doses of neighborhood nature: the benefits for mental health of living with nature*, Cox DTC, Shanahan DF, Hudson HL, Plummer KE, Siriwardena GM, Fuller RA, Anderson K, Hancock S, Gaston KJ (2017), *BioScience*, vol. 67,2: 147-155: doi.org/10.1093/biosci/biw173

24. *The power of support from companion animals for people living with mental health problems: a systematic review and narrative synthesis of the evidence*, Brooks HL, Rushton K, Lovell K et al (2018), *BMC Psychiatry*, vol. 18,31: doi.org/10.1186/s12888-018-1613-2

25. *Using and disclosing patient information for direct care, Ethical guidance for doctors*, General Medical Council (2021): www.gmc-uk.org/ethical-guidance/ethical-guidance-for-doctors/confidentiality/using-and-disclosing-patient-information-for-direct-care
26. *Borderline personality disorder recognition and management, Clinical Guideline CG78*, National Institute for Clinical Excellence (NICE) (2021): www.nice.org.uk/guidance/cg78/ifp/chapter/Glossary
27. *Post-traumatic stress disorder, Guideline N6116*, National Institute for Clinical Excellence (NICE) (2018): www.nice.org.uk/guidance/ng116/chapter/recommendations
28. *Mental Capacity Act*, HM Government (2005): www.legislation.gov.uk/ukpga/2005/9/contents

TriggerHub is one of the most elite and scientifically proven forms of mental health intervention

Trigger Publishing is the leading independent mental health and wellbeing publisher in the UK and US. Clinical and scientific research conducted by assistant professor Dr Kristin Kosyluk and her highly acclaimed team in the Department of Mental Health Law & Policy at the University of South Florida (USF), as well as complementary research by her peers across the US, has independently verified the power of lived experience as a core component in achieving mental health prosperity. Specifically, the lived experiences contained within our bibliotherapeutic books are intrinsic elements in reducing stigma, making those with poor mental health feel less alone, providing the privacy they need to heal, ensuring they know the essential steps to kick-start their own journeys to recovery, and providing hope and inspiration when they need it most.

Delivered through TriggerHub, our unique online portal and accompanying smartphone app, we make our library of bibliotherapeutic titles and other vital resources accessible to individuals and organizations anywhere, at any time and with complete privacy, a crucial element of recovery. As such, TriggerHub is the primary recommendation across the UK and US for the delivery of lived experiences.

At Trigger Publishing and TriggerHub, we proudly lead the way in making the unseen become seen. We are dedicated to humanizing mental health, breaking stigma and challenging outdated societal values to create real action and impact. Find out more about our world-leading work with lived experience and bibliotherapy via triggerhub.com, or by joining us on:

🐦 @triggerhub_

🅕 @triggerhub.org

📷 @triggerhub_

Printed in the USA
CPSIA information can be obtained
at www.ICGtesting.com
JSHW031710140824
68134JS00038B/3627